Pancreatitis

Essential Pancreatitis Guide with 100 Recipes and a

30 Day Meal Plan for Better Health

Richard Smith Johnson

Introduction

The pancreas is a vital organ that's found in our abdomen and plays the role of converting the food you eat into fuel that can be used by your body's cells for energy. However, the pancreas is one of the organs that we don't really pay much attention to, unless we start falling sick and on a visit to the doctor, we are told that the pancreas is not working properly.

If you are reading this book chances are that you, a friend or relative has had a painful encounter with pancreatitis. This book is going to help you understand what pancreatitis is, the fact that it's not a life sentence and how you can beat it.

However, it is important that you understand that beating it is going to require a fundamental change in your life. You can take two approaches; one is the band aid approach that will see you get some temporary relief from pain or two, the approach of going to the root cause of the problem and following the recommended treatment by a medical doctor.

As with most diseases, you will realize, as you read on, that it all starts with the food you eat. There is a common phrase that is used in the world of computers and it goes, "Garbage in, Garbage out." If we use the same analogy when it comes to what we eat, it simply means that if you follow a healthy diet that comprises of natural, whole foods, then you will have a healthy body as you constantly nourish it with exactly what it needs. On the other hand if most of the food you eat is processed and fast food, which more often than not contains very little nutrition, then you can expect to have a body that is constantly under attack from disease.

However, it is important to point that some causes of pancreatitis may well be out our control in the case of hyperactive immune function.

This book is going to focus on using nutrition to help your body naturally heal itself and rehabilitate the pancreas to better health as you will see with the introductory section as well as the recipe section. However, please note that this is a self-published book and it is my recommendation that you first see a doctor and also do your own research alongside what I will be sharing in this guide. Everything in this book is based on my research and experience with the disease.

Without further ado, put on your glasses and let's take the first step in this beautiful journey!

The Pancreas

As mentioned earlier, the pancreas is located in your abdomen. It serves two primary functions: an endocrine function that sees it regulate your blood sugar levels and an exocrine function that helps in the digestive process.

- **Endocrine function**

Aside from being a digestive gland, the pancreas is also an endocrine gland. The portion of the pancreas responsible for the endocrine function is known as the endocrine component and is made of islet cells. These cells secrete two important hormones into your bloodstream and these are glucagon ad insulin.

Insulin

Insulin is formed in beta cells and interestingly only has approximately 8 minutes of half life in your blood. The main stimulus for the release of insulin is elevated blood glucose levels. Insulin then helps the cells in your body that need glucose for energy to ingest it faster which leads to a drop in your blood glucose value.

Insulin also helps in the process of storing excess glucose that the body cannot immediately use for energy.

Glucagon

This hormone is secreted in the alpha cells of your pancreas. When you have low blood glucose levels, glucagon starts the process of glycogenolysis which is literally the breaking down of glycogen (stored glucose) into glucose, availing it for use by your cells for energy. Glucagon inhibits the process of storing glucose for energy which in effect leads to a rise in blood glucose levels.

Maintaining the proper balance of blood sugar is critical to the proper functioning of vital organs such as the heart, brain, kidneys and liver.

- **Exocrine function**

The pancreas has exocrine glands that secrete enzymes that play a very important role in the digestive process. These include chymotrypsin and trypsin that help digest protein, lipase that helps in the breakdown of fats and amylase that helps in the breakdown of carbs.

Once food moves from your mouth to your stomach, these enzymes are released into an intricate set of ducts that join the bile duct in the first part of your small intestines (duodenum) which help digest the food.

Diseases That Affect the Pancreas

There are three main diseases that affect the pancreas, and these are: pancreatitis, precancerous pancreas conditions and pancreatic cancer. Each of these may present unique symptoms and may require different forms of treatment.

Pancreatitis

This is inflammation of the pancreas that occurs as a result of the pancreatic juices accumulating beyond normal levels and beginning to digest the pancreas itself. At onset, pancreatitis manifests as sharp pains that can last for a number of days before going away. With more progression, pancreatitis may develop into a chronic condition that lasts for years.

Precancerous pancreas conditions

Medics and scientists have not been able to establish the exact cause of cancer of the pancreas. What is known is a number of risk factors such as genetic cancer syndromes, cigarette smoking or a family history of pancreatic cancer. There are additional precancerous conditions that also increase the risk of cancer and these are lesions that form on the pancreas such as Pancreatic Intraepithelial Neoplastic (PanIN) AND Intraductal Papillary Mucinous Neoplasms (IPMNs).

Pancreatic Cancer

Pancreatic Adenocarcinoma is the most common form of pancreatic cancer which grows on the exocrine glands of the pancreas. Endocrine tumors are not common and only account for less than 5 percent of all pancreatic cancer cases that are reported.

Understanding Pancreatitis

We have so far established that pancreatitis occurs as a result of inflammation that is caused by the pancreatic enzymes starting to digest the pancreas, which shouldn't happen. To get a better understanding of this condition, we will start by looking at how your pancreas should function under normal circumstances. When you put food in your mouth, a signal is sent to your stomach alerting it that there is food coming through and to thus prepare all the digestive system components. As food goes down your digestive tract, enzymes are released that help in the digestion process. For example, if you eat a delicious piece of steak, the enzymes that are released (chymotrypsin and trypsin) are so potent that they devour the meat very quickly.

Our bodies need these enzymes to be this strong otherwise it wouldn't be possible for you to enjoy a juicy steak or chops. Under normal circumstances, we don't pay much thought to what happens to the food we eat from the moment we put it in our moths to the moment we poop. The truth is that the pancreas plays a pivotal role in the digestive process as it's responsible for the synthesis and release of these enzymes.

When you develop pancreatitis, the secreted enzymes that are normally released into the first part of the small intestine (duodenum), get triggered whilst still in the pancreas. Question is, if these enzymes are created in the pancreas, why does the pancreas get hurt? Shouldn't it be able to handle these enzymes? Well, the above-mentioned process may have oversimplified the process of enzymatic release in relation to digestion. What happens is that these enzymes do not get triggered until they mix with other digestive chemicals, a process that takes place in the duodenum.

However, this does not hold when pancreatitis occurs, and the enzymes are triggered whilst in the pancreas therein beginning to digest the pancreas. When this happens, we now have a huge problem inside the pancreas. The body being well equipped to stop attacks even that which is caused by its own components, activates inflammation. When pancreatic cells get in contact with the prematurely triggered enzymes, its blood vessel and tissues get inflamed as they are being literally digested and they are trying to 'heal' themselves. However, if this persists the self-digestion that the pancreatic tissues and vessels begin to bleed and the pancreas starts to lose function and the enzymes start leaking to other parts of the digestive system, a process that results in a lot of pain. Pancreatitis on onset has been described as a very sharp and burning pain that is felt right below the ribs or between your abdomen and back. To some, they have described the pain as having thought that they were experiencing a heart attack. Some have fainted while others have had severe bouts of vomiting because of pancreatitis.

Pancreatitis can occur as a sudden attack, in some cases it could last for a couple for days while in others it can go for weeks or even months, solely depending on what is the trigger and the health of the patient in question. When a person first experiences pancreatitis, there is a chance that this could recur and it is important that they seek medical help in order to determine the cause and what to do to ensure it does not happen again.

Symptoms of Pancreatitis

Most people who suffer or have suffered from pancreatitis, be it acute or chronic, have sited pain the left upper abdominals. For people with chronic pancreatitis, inflammation may be spotted on diagnostic imaging scans.

The other common symptoms of pancreatitis are:

- Sever nausea and vomiting
- Pain that seems to wrap the upper abdomen all the way to the back
- Bloating with a swollen tummy
- Tenderness on the upper abdomen
- Severe hiccups
- Unexplained weight loss
- Fever
- Fatty stool (steatorrhea), common in people with chronic pancreatitis

Steatorrhea is a sign that your body is not being able to absorb most of the nutrients you ingest and this is a sign that your pancreas is not releasing enough enzymes needed in the process of digestion.

Types of pancreatitis

There are two main types of pancreatitis and these are acute and chronic pancreatitis. We also have necrotizing pancreatitis that stems from very severe cases of acute pancreatitis. We are going to delve into each type to get a better understanding of each type.

Acute Pancreatitis

Pancreatitis is the main cause for the greater percentage of all gastrointestinal hospital admissions. This is according to the National Institute of Diabetes, Digestive and Kidney Diseases. As mentioned earlier, acute pancreatitis occurs very suddenly. It manifests as auto-digestion of your pancreatic tissue and this is caused by the premature release of zymogens. It is very common in adults and often requires immediate medical attention owing to how painful it is and for most people, they don't understand what's going on and some actually think they are experiencing a heart attack. For some people the pain occurs in the upper abdomen and spreads to the back in a belt-like fashion. Some patients with acute pancreatitis develop a false cyst that spontaneously appears and regresses. Tenderness in the upper abdomen, bruising around the trunk area as well as a reddened face are some of the symptoms that stand out. It is important that you and your doctor find out the trigger for the acute pancreatitis. If it's alcohol or cigarettes; the next course of action will include you quitting alcohol or cigarettes in order to prevent another flare up or progression into chronic pancreatitis.

Necrotizing Pancreatitis

Necrosis refers to the dying of cells. Very severe cases of acute pancreatitis could lead to some parts of the pancreas dying. This often occurs when acute pancreatitis is not addressed in good time. For example, one could take pain medication when they start experiencing the 'wrap around' upper abdominal pain that is associated with pancreatitis. The problem with this approach is that it is possible to mask the pain for a couple of days. However, the root of the problem is not addressed meaning inflammation of the pancreas becomes even more sever and by the time the patient is seeking medical help, part of the pancreas will have already started dying.

Diagnosis is often done using a CT scan or an abdominal ultrasound. The doctor may also take a sample of the dead pancreas tissue to check for infection. In the case of infection, the patient will be prescribed for antibiotics and in some cases the dead tissue will have to be removed.

Infection of necrotizing pancreatitis increases the risk of death and this is something that needs to be addressed as soon as it's diagnosed.

Chronic Pancreatitis

As the name suggests, chronic pancreatitis refers to inflammation of the pancreas that stems from several bouts of acute pancreatitis or pancreatitis that has consistently occurred over a long period of time. Patients of chronic pancreatitis often have permanent damage on their pancreas that involves a lot of scar tissue formation from the continued inflammation.

Alcohol abuse accounts for 70 percent of all chronic pancreatitis cases. Genetic and autoimmune conditions such as cystic fibrosis can also lead to chronic pancreatitis. It is important for people suffering from chronic pancreatitis to be able to identify the root cause of the disease, with the help of their doctors. Once this has been established, it is now possible to implement a plan that will help reduce symptoms and also help the body to try and start healing itself.

Causes of Pancreatitis

In 20 percent of the cases, there is no known cause of a pancreatitis attack. The most common triggers are diabetes, gallstones and alcohol. In the case of alcohol, the solution is as simple as not taking alcohol anymore. It's a choice between health and the pain and trauma brought about by pancreatitis. In the case of pancreatitis that has been triggered by gallstones, the solution involves first dealing with the gallstones. For diabetes, treatment involves normalizing insulin levels and treatment for diabetes.

a. Diabetes

A greater percentage of patients with pancreatitis also suffer from diabetes. Since insulin is the hormone tasked with the role of decreasing blood sugar levels, a deficiency in insulin leads to hyperglycemia- an increase in blood glucose levels and glycosuria – elevated glucose excretion in a patient's urine.

Type 1 diabetes

Patients with type 1 diabetes suffer from insulin deficiency that comes from the destruction of beta cells by antibodies. Patients are usually younger than those with type 2 diabetes with most ranging from 15 to 25 years. Type 1 diabetes patients exogenously take in insulin all through their lives.

Type 2 diabetes

Insulin deficiency occurs in patients as a result of the peripheral cells being resistant to insulin. Type 2 diabetes mostly affects adults and thus the term *adult-onset diabetes.* Treatment involves a healthy, natural and balanced diet, loss of extra weight, physical exercise and oral type 2 diabetes medication.

Why are people with diabetes at risk of getting pancreatitis?

- Elevated triglyceride levels

Diabetes patients usually have increased levels of triglycerides (a type of fat) in their blood. Both type 1 and type 2 diabetes patients can have hypertriglyceridemia and when it's too high can lead to pancreatitis. Lowering these fats can help prevent pancreatitis and this can be done by maintaining normal levels of blood sugar by monitoring insulin levels.

- Auto-immune attacks

Type 1 diabetes is an autoimmune condition and as such can leave patients exposed to other forms of autoimmune attacks which include variations of pancreatitis.

- Gallstones

Diabetes patients stand a higher chance of having gallstones and as we are going to see in a short while, gallstones are one of the common causes of pancreatitis.

b. Alcohol

A greater percentage of pancreatitis cases are attributed to alcohol abuse. Alcohol abuse in this case refers to years of excessive alcohol intake. how alcohol impacts the pancreas is yet to be fully established especially its link to pancreatitis attacks. What is known is that alcohol abuse leads to inflammation of the pancreas.

c. Gallstones

These are hardened deposits of digestive fluids that are found in the gall bladder that can clog bile ducts thus inhibiting the flow of pancreatic enzymes. In the case of gallstones, the best course of action to take it to naturally detoxify your gall bladder.

d. Surgery in the stomach, lungs or heart where the blood supply to the pancreas was temporarily cut off
e. Cystic fibrosis
f. Trauma to the abdomen
g. Medication such as sulfanomides, nonsteroidal anti-inflammatory drugs, azathioprine, corticosteroids and certain antibiotics. Always take these drugs under your doctor's advisement.
h. High calcium and triglyceride levels in the blood
i. Infections such as hepatitis, mumps and rubella

Gall Bladder Detox

The aim of a gall bladder detox is to treat gallstones for those who may already have them or protect a person from getting them in the first place.

The gall bladder is a small pocket that stores the bile secreted by the liver and bile helps your body digest fat and other foods that are difficult to process in a more effective manner. Gallstones are solid deposits that form in the gall bladder and can cause pancreatitis, and extreme pain if they block a duct in the gall bladder.

How to Detox your Gall Bladder

- Include apples in your detox diet

When doing a gall bladder detox, look for tart apples such as Granny Smith apples and blend them in your detox juice, add to a salad or eat as is. Also add apple cider vinegar, that is unfiltered (it will have the words 'with the mother' on the bottle) to your drinking water to help cleanse both your liver and gall bladder. Additionally, you can use apple cider vinegar to make salad dressing for your salads. However, avoid drinking it raw as it can be quite corrosive.

- Drink herbal teas and a lot of water to help flush out toxins

Most herbal teas have great detoxing attributes that are attributed to their antioxidant and hydrating properties. Milk thistle, red clover and stinging nettle are especially good for digestion and cleansing your liver and gall bladder.

- Avoid gall bladder inflammatory foods

Meats, dairy, seeds and nuts have been shown to cause gall bladder problem when eaten excessively. During your gall bladder detox, it's advisable to avoid these foods and once you are done with the cleanse, you can start re-introducing them little by little. Remember to take everything in moderation.

Processed sugars and alcohol have also been shown to inhibit the gall bladder from processing toxins and bile.

Your diet should feature a lot of organic greens, healthy fats and a lot of water.

- Get adequate sleep

Eight hours of uninterrupted sleep is ideal for all your internal processes to continue without getting interrupted. This will help the natural detoxification process to take place.

A gall bladder detox is very similar to a liver detox as the gall bladder's functionality is made possible by the liver. It is therefore possible to reap liver detox benefits from a gall bladder detox and vice versa. Try both of them and then you can switch to the one that worked best for you.

Diagnosis and Treatment of Pancreatitis

- **Diagnosis**

There is no one sure fire way to diagnose pancreatitis. In fact, diagnosis usually involves a series of tests and these include:

1. CT scans to check for gallstones as well as inflammation
2. An endoscopic ultrasound to check for any blockages in the bile and pancreatic ducts as well as inflammation.
3. **Lab tests**: elevated levels of lipase and amylase. When these are three times the normal levels, it can be an indication of acute pancreatitis.

   Increased AP-Alkaline phosphates, CGT- gamma-glutamyl transferase, SGOT – serum glutamic oxaloacetic transaminaseare usually indicative of a bile duct obstruction as the cause for pancreatitis.

4. Abdominal ultrasound to check for gallstones and surrounding inflammation
5. An MRI to check for any anomaly in the pancreas, gallbladder, bile and pancreas ducts
6. Stool tests to check for steatorrhea. Presence of high levels of fat is an indication that not enough enzymes are being released to help in the digestion of fats

- **Medical Treatment**

Fasting

A nothing by mouth treatment regimen is recommended for a patient with acute pancreatitis. The reason of prescribed fasting is to rest the pancreas and stop any enzymatic secretions and the digestive function as well.

1. Slow and monitored fluid therapy with electrolytes to avoid an electrolyte imbalance and dehydration. This is especially important for patients with severe vomiting and diarrhea.
2. Gallstone removal is the next step. Surgery should be done in cases where conservative approaches to remove gallstones do not work.
3. Natural Treatment

Natural treatment is advised to help manage symptoms after proper medical diagnosis and treatment has taken place. Diet and lifestyle changes play a very important role when it comes to preventing of symptoms. It is important to note that natural treatment should only be administered during the recessive phase of pancreatitis. Some of the natural remedies you can employ include:

Embrace A Natural and Healthy Diet

Diet is very important when it comes to prevention, management, and recovery from pancreatitis.

Foods to eliminate:

    a. Avoid all foods that contain allergens such as wheat, dairy, soy, processed food additives and preservatives

    b. Reduce or completely avoid foods containing trans-fats

    c. Avoid taking stimulants such as alcohol, tobacco and caffeine

What to eat

- Add healthy oils such coconut oil, avocado oil and olive oil to your meals
- Eat foods that are rich in iron such as lentils, 70 percent dark chocolate, pastured beef liver and spirulina
- Eat anti-oxidant rich foods that will help reduce inflammation such as blueberries, bell peppers, tomatoes and cherries
- Eat a low fat diet that focuses on fresh veggies, fruit, whole grains and lean proteins
- Eat food that's as close as possible to plants or animals. In short, steer away from processed foods

1. **Eliminate nutrient deficiencies**
   Your doctor will test your blood for any deficiencies and if present alter your diet to eliminate these deficiencies. Your doctor will also advise you on whether it's necessary for you to take supplements.

2. **Seek alternative pain management therapies**
   After you've been diagnosed with pancreatitis and have already embarked on medication to help manage and reduce symptoms, you may choose to explore natural therapies to help manage the pain.
   These therapies are meant to help you find Zen and to also help your body heal itself heal faster. These include meditation, yoga, acupuncture and relaxation exercises.

Feed Your Pancreas

Cruciferous and leafy green vegetables

Veggies are some of the best gut cleansing foods because of their high fiber content that plays a crucial role in the waste elimination process. Additionally, they are also rich in vitamins, antioxidants and minerals. Spinach, kale, broccoli, cauliflower, collard greens and cabbages should always be part of your diet, especially when you want to keep your whole digestive system running smoothly.

Eat your veggies Raw, or very lightly steamed for you to get the maximum nutrition from this veggies.

Combine then with healthy fats such as avocado or olive oil to maximize the absorption of nutrients from these vegetables.

Probiotics

These are healthy bacteria that help in the digestion process. Fermented foods are very rich in probiotics. Go for organic and natural probiotics such as kimchi, yogurt, kefir, sauerkraut, kombucha and miso. These together with enzymes from the pancreas will help the digestive process work efficiently.

Chia seeds

Chia seeds are a very rich source of omega-3 fats that are highly anti-inflammatory. This is an important benefit especially for an inflamed pancreas as it can help reduce inflammation.

Drink plenty of water

The more water that goes into your gut, the healthier it is. Water helps remove toxins from the gut as well as helping food get digested faster. Therefore combine your healthy diet with increased water intake. You should aim for half your body weight in ounces.

Wild caught fish

Fish is high in omea-3 fatty acids which that help reduce inflammation. Wild caught fish is more organic than farmed fish and has been shown to have higher levels of omega-3 fats. Part of this is attributed to the fact that farmed fish are primarily fed on grains which are not as nutritious as worms and other sea life that wild fish feed on in lakes and seas.

Natural fruit and veggies

Dark leafy greens provide your body with Vitamins A&C, iron, calcium and folate which boost your body's metabolism. Kale, Brussels sprouts, watercress, spinach, rocket and broccoli are full of heart healthy nutrients. Fruits such as grapefruit, oranges, berries, pineapple are also a good way to feed your body with healthy nutrients.

Whole grains and pulses

With a high iron and protein contents, whole grains and pulses boost gut health.They also lower the risk of diabetes and heart disease.

When it comes to food, remember that everything should be done in moderation. However, avoid processed foods that are high in unhealthy fats and very high in processed sugar.

Conclusion

The human body as made in such a way that it could take of all its vital processes such as digestion on its own without outside help. It was so efficiently designed that it could fix any problem with any of its organs without outside intervention.

Unfortunately, with the evolution of what we eat from what our ancestors ate has rendered the body incapable of keeping up with all its processes without breaking down.

This book explores one vital organ and what it is responsible for, what affects it and ways in which we can be able to keep it healthy. The first step is going back to the diet that was followed by our ancestors. As simple as eating healthy and natural foods. Feed your body with food that will nourish it and not make it seek.

Am confident that you have been able to get important information on how to keep your pancreas healthy and how to manage any symptom of pancreatitis. Enjoy the recipes on our food section that have been specifically designed to help you manage and prevent symptoms of pancreatitis.

Remember to share with friends and family so we are able to help so many people who are living in the anguish of pancreatitis pain.

All the best as you embrace a healthier life that is now more informed!

30-DAY PANCREATITIS DIET MEAL PLAN

Please make sure that the calorie intake is sufficient for your body.

Day	Breakfast	AM SNACK	Lunch	PM SNACK	Dinner
DAY 1	Low Fat Chilli & Onion Omelet	1 Cup Fruity Detox Tea	Spiced Sweet Potato and Spring Onion Salad	Amaranth Pop Corns	Beef & Sweet Potato Enchilada Casserole
DAY 2	Buckwheat Pancakes with Elderberries	1 Cup Turmeric Detox Tea	Healthy Millet Lettuce Wraps	Gingery Apple & Spinach Juice	Yummy Chicken and Sweet Potato Stew
DAY 3	Buckwheat Cereal with Red Onions & Mushrooms	1 Cup Lemon, Ginger & Turmeric Detox Tea	Healthy Salad with Hot Berry Dressing	Beef & Millet Stuffed Peppers	Delicious Buckwheat with Mushrooms & Green Onions
DAY 4	Superfood Overnight Oats	1 Cup Active Weight Loss Tea	Warm Bean Soup with Whole-Wheat Tortilla Chips	Chilled Pineapple-Ginger Ale	Healthy Fried Brown Rice with Peas & Prawns
DAY 5	Low Fat Omelets with Mushrooms & Veggies	1 Cup Apple Cider Detox Tea	Low Fat Salad with Ginger & Lemon Dressing	Spiced Apple Crisps	Delicious Buckwheat with Mushrooms & Green Onions
DAY 6	Healthy Amaranth Porridge	1 Cup Mint and Parsley Fat Burning Tea	Cauliflower & Broccoli Soup	Ginger Berry Pineapple Drink	Asparagus Quinoa & Steak Bowl

DAY 7	Spiced Mushroom Egg Scramble	1 Cup Fruity Detox Tea	Green Salad with Beets & Edamame	Crispy Lemon- Chili Roasted Kale	Yummy Chicken and Sweet Potato Stew
DAY 8	Healthy Brown Rice Breakfast Bowl	1 Cup Lemon, Ginger & Turmeric Detox Tea	Winter Savory Soup	Carrot & Celery Juice	Seared Lemon Steak with Vegetables Stir-Fry
DAY 9	Spiced Egg Frittata	1 Cup Turmeric Detox Tea	Low Fat Vegetable & Orange Salad with Citrus Ginger Dressing	Healthy Taro Chips	Delicious Low Fat Chicken Curry
DAY 10	Healthy Buckwheat, Millet and Amaranth Porridge	1 Cup Fruity Detox Tea	Stir-Fried Mushrooms & Spinach with Golden Onions	Berry Freshness	Vegetable Tabbouleh
DAY 11	Mushrooms, Boiled Eggs & Veggie Breakfast Bowl	1 Cup Lemon, Ginger & Turmeric Detox Tea	Green Bean, Broccoli & Carrot Salad	Healthy Taro Chips	Grilled Chicken Breast with Non-Fat Yogurt
DAY 12	Citrus Superfood Breakfast Smoothie Bowl	1 Cup Active Weight Loss Tea	Spiced Lentils & Brown Rice Dish	Cucumber Aloe Vera Drink	Peppered Steak with Cherry Tomatoes
DAY 13	Low Fat Omelets with Mushrooms & Veggies	1 Cup Apple Cider Detox Tea	Stir-Fried Beef, Shiitake Mushrooms and Peppers	Sweet Spiced Mango-Mint Lassi	Vegetable Tabbouleh

DAY 14	Ginger Almond Berry Smoothie Bowl	1 Cup Mint and Parsley Fat Burning Tea	Spiced Carrot Soup	Refreshing Cucumber Citrus Juice	Tilapia with Mushroom Sauce
DAY 15	Low Fat Sweet Potato & Turkey Breakfast Casserole	1 Cup Lemon, Ginger & Turmeric Detox Tea	Superfood Nutty Salad with Hot Citrus Dressing	Chia Seed Millet Flour Cake	Beef & Sweet Potato Enchilada Casserole
DAY 16	Lemon Blueberry Almond Smoothie	1 Cup Fruity Detox Tea	Spiced Vegetable Indian Soup	Kale & Apple Juice	Ginger Chicken with Veggies
DAY 17	Buckwheat Pancakes with Elderberries	1 Cup Active Weight Loss Tea	Raw Vegetable & Papaya Salad	Low-Carb Cassava Crepes	Asparagus Quinoa & Steak Bowl
DAY 18	The Ultimate Detox Smoothie	1 Cup Turmeric Detox Tea	Spiced Healthy Cauliflower Bowl	Celery Pineapple Juice	Hot Lemon Prawns
DAY 19	Healthy Buckwheat, Millet and Amaranth Porridge	1 Cup Fruity Detox Tea	Spiced Sweet Potato and Spring Onion Salad	Vinegar & Salt Kale Chips	Delicious Low Fat Chicken Curry

DAY 20	Low Fat Greek Yogurt with Acai Berry Granola	1 Cup Active Weight Loss Tea	Detox Lemon Leek & Broccoli Soup	Apple & Citrus Beet Juice	Delicious Chicken Tikka Skewers
DAY 21	Spiced Egg Frittata	1 Cup Turmeric Detox Tea	Green Bean, Broccoli & Carrot Salad	Crispy Lemon- Chili Roasted Kale	Healthy Fried Brown Rice with Peas & Prawns
DAY 22	Healthy Millet Porridge	1 Cup Lemon, Ginger & Turmeric Detox Tea	Low Fat Lemon & Turmeric Lentil Soup	Hot Ginger Cucumber & Beet Juice	Grilled Chicken with Salad Wrap
DAY 23	Low Fat Chilli & Onion Omelet	1 Cup Apple Cider Detox Tea	Vitamin-Rich Salad	Spiced Apple Crisps	Seared Lemon Steak with Vegetables Stir-Fry
DAY 24	Wholesome Buckwheat Pancakes	1 Cup Active Weight Loss Tea	Chickpea Salad Wrap	Red Detox Juice	Authentic and Easy Shrimp Curry
DAY 25	Low Fat Sweet Potato & Turkey Breakfast Casserole	1 Cup Lemon, Ginger & Turmeric Detox Tea	Stir-Fried Beef, Shiitake Mushrooms and Peppers	Beef & Millet Stuffed Peppers	Healthy Black Bean Chili
DAY 26	Citrus Turmeric Smoothie	1 Cup Mint and Parsley Fat Burning Tea	Warm Bean Soup with Whole-Wheat Tortilla Chips	Chia Seed Millet Flour Cake	Spiced Almond Milk Lentil Stew

DAY 27	Mushrooms, Boiled Eggs & Veggie Breakfast Bowl	1 Cup Fruity Detox Tea	Low Fat Vegetable & Orange Salad with Citrus Ginger Dressing	Spiced Ginger Citrus Juice	Delicious Buckwheat with Mushrooms & Green Onions
DAY 28	Chai Spiced Greek Yogurt Parfait with Fresh Fruits	1 Cup Active Weight Loss Tea	Warm Bean Soup with Whole-Wheat Tortilla Chips	Amaranth Pop Corns	Hot Lemon Prawns
DAY 29	Spiced Mushroom Egg Scramble	1 Cup Turmeric Detox Tea	Healthy Salad with Hot Berry Dressing	Ginger Citrus Asparagus Body Cleanser	Beef & Sweet Potato Enchilada Casserole
DAY 30	Buckwheat Pancakes with Elderberries	1 Cup Lemon, Ginger & Turmeric Detox Tea	Healthy Millet Lettuce Wraps	Healthy Taro Chips	Yummy Chicken and Sweet Potato Stew

PANCREATITIS RECIPES

BREAKFAST RECIPES

MORNING TEAS

1. Lemon, Ginger & Turmeric Detox Tea

Yield: 2 Servings
Total Time: 10 Minutes
Prep Time: 10 Minutes
Cook Time: 20 Minutes

Ingredients

- 6 bags of green tea
- 2 cups water
- 1 cup chopped fresh ginger
- 3 cinnamon sticks
- 1 teaspoon ground turmeric
- 1 teaspoon cayenne pepper
- 1 cup fresh lemon juice

Directions

Add chopped ginger and green tea bags to a pan of water and bring to a rolling boil. Lower heat and simmer for about 10 minutes. Add in turmeric, cinnamon stick, and cayenne pepper and cook for another 10 minutes. remove the pan from heat and let cool before straining. Stir in lemon juice and refrigerate for at least 1 hour or until chilled.

Enjoy!

Nutritional Information per Serving:

Calories: 194; Total Fat: 3.9 g; Carbs: 37.1 g; Dietary Fiber: 8.2 g; Protein: 4.2 g; Cholesterol: 0 mg; Sodium: 46 mg

2. Active Weight Loss Tea

Yield: 2 Servings
Total Time: 2 Hours 30 Minutes
Prep Time: 10 Minutes
Cook Time: 1 Hour 20 Minutes

Ingredients

- 4 cups hot water
- 1-inch ginger root, thinly sliced
- 2 cinnamon sticks
- 4 green tea bags
- ½ cup freshly squeezed lemon juice

Optional:

- Raw honey, to taste

Directions

Add the hot water to a large pot over high heat and add the cinnamon stick and sliced ginger. Bring to a boil then turn off the heat. Add the tea bags and lemon juice and let the tea steep.

You can drink this tea as is or sweeten it with some raw honey.

Sip on this tea first thing in the morning, before your breakfast and last thing before you sleep for maximum fat burning benefits.

Nutritional Information per Serving:

Calories: 47; Total Fat: 1.2 g; Carbs: 7.5 g; Dietary Fiber: 3.1 g; Protein: 1.3 g; Cholesterol: 0 mg; Sodium: 54 mg

3. Fruity Detox Tea

Yield: 1 Serving
Total Time: 2 Hours 30 Minutes
Prep Time: 10 Minutes
Cook Time: 1 Hour 20 Minutes

Ingredients

- 2 cucumber slices
- 1 lemon slice
- 2 strawberries, thinly sliced
- 1 green tea bag
- 1 tsp. raw honey
- 1 cup boiling hot water

Directions

Add the tea bag to the cup of water and let steep until it cools completely. Stir in all the remaining ingredients and you are ready to drink.

You can add some ice cubes, if you like your tea super chilled.

Nutritional Information per Serving:

Calories: 49; Total Fat: 0.2 g; Carbs: 12 g; Dietary Fiber: 1.2 g; Protein: 0.9 g; Cholesterol: 0 mg; Sodium: 3 mg

4. Turmeric Detox Tea

Yield: 4 Servings
Total Time: 2 Hours 30 Minutes
Prep Time: 10 Minutes

Ingredients

- 2 whole cinnamon sticks
- ¼ tsp. cayenne pepper
- 3-inch ginger root, finely chopped
- ½ tsp. turmeric powder
- 4 fresh lemons
- 4 cups water

Directions

Add the hot water to a large pot over medium to high heat. Stir in the chopped ginger and bring to a boil. Lower the heat and let simmer for 8 minutes. Add in the turmeric, cinnamon sticks and cayenne and continue simmering for 10 minutes. Turn off the heat and let it cool. Squeeze in fresh lemon juice.

You can either drink this warm or chilled.

Nutritional Information per Serving:

Calories: 89; Total Fat: 1.5 g; Carbs: 36.1 g; Dietary Fiber: 10.2 g; Protein: 4.2 g; Cholesterol: 0 mg; Sodium: 37 mg

5. Apple Cider Detox Tea

Yield: 1 Serving
Total Time: 2 Hours 30 Minutes
Prep Time: 10 Minutes

Ingredients

- 2 tbsp. organic apple cider vinegar
- ¼ tsp. cinnamon powder
- ½ tsp. ginger powder
- 1 pinch cayenne powder
- 2 tbsp. freshly squeezed lemon juice
- 1 tsp. raw honey
- 1 glass hot water

Directions

Combine all ingredients in a mug and drink hot, warm or chilled.

Nutritional Information per Serving:

Calories: 39; Total Fat: 0.3 g; Carbs: 7.5 g; Dietary Fiber: 0.3 g; Protein: 0.4 g; Cholesterol: 0 mg; Sodium: 8 mg

6. Mint and Parsley Fat Burning Tea

Yield: 1 Serving
Total Time: 2 Hours 30 Minutes
Prep Time: 10 Minutes

Ingredients

- 1 tsp. freshly chopped mint
- 1 tsp. freshly chopped parsley
- 1 cup boiling hot water
- 2 tbsp. freshly squeezed lemon juice

Directions

Stir in the mint and parsley in the hot water and let stand for 5 minutes.

Stir in the lemon juice and enjoy!

Nutritional Information per Serving:

Calories: 9; Total Fat: 0.3 g; Carbs: 0.9 g; Dietary Fiber: 0.3 g; Protein: 0.3 g; Cholesterol: 0 mg; Sodium: 15 mg

BREAKFAST RECIPES

7. Buckwheat Pancakes with Elderberries

Yield: 4 Servings
Total Time: 26 Minutes
Prep Time: 10 Minutes
Cook Time: 16 Minutes

Ingredients

- 1 teaspoon coconut oil
- 1 cup almond milk
- 1 cup ground buckwheat flour
- ½ teaspoon chili powder
- ¼ teaspoon turmeric powder
- teaspoon salt
- ¼ teaspoon black pepper
- ½ inch ginger, grated
- 1 serrano pepper, minced
- 1 handful cilantro, chopped
- ½ red onion, chopped
- 1 cup fresh elderberries to serve

Directions

In a bowl, combine together buckwheat, almond milk, and spices until well combined; stir in red onion, cilantro, ginger and Serrano pepper until well blended.

Melt coconut oil in a saucepan over medium low heat; add about one quarter of a cup of batter and spread out on the pan.

Cook the pancakes for about 4 minutes per side or until golden brown. Transfer to a plate and keep warm; repeat with the remaining batter and oil.

Top the pancakes with fresh elderberries and fold into wraps. Serve with a glass of freshly squeezed orange juice.

Nutritional Information per Serving:

Calories: 386; Total Fat: 6.3 g; Carbs: 20.5 g; Dietary Fiber: 3.5g; Sugars: 3.2 g; Protein: 4.1 g; Cholesterol: 0 mg; Sodium: 596 mg

8. Healthy Amaranth Porridge

Yield: 2 Servings
Total Time: 40 Minutes
Prep Time: 10 Minutes
Cook Time: 30 Minutes

Ingredients

- ½ cup amaranth
- 1 ½ cups water
- ¼ cup almond milk
- 1 teaspoon stevia
- ¼ teaspoon sea salt

Directions

In a pan, combine water, salt and amaranth and bring to a boil; cover and simmer for about 30 minutes and then stir in milk and stevia and cook, stirring until the porridge in creamy. Serve right away.

Nutritional Information per Serving:

Calories: 190; Total Fat: 3.8 g; Net Carbs: 27.7 g; Dietary Fiber: 4.8 g; Sugars: 0.8 g; Protein: 7.3 g; Cholesterol: 0 mg; Sodium: 287 mg

9. Healthy Brown Rice Breakfast Bowl

Yield: 4 Servings
Total Time: 20 Minutes
Prep Time: 10 Minutes
Cook Time: 10 Minutes

Ingredients

- 2 cups cooked brown rice
- 1/2 cup unsweetened almond milk
- 1 teaspoon liquid stevia
- 1 tablespoon almond butter
- 1 apple, diced
- 2 dates, chopped
- 1/2 teaspoon cinnamon

Directions

Combine almond oil, almond butter, stevia, apple and dates in a saucepan; bring to a gentle boil and then cook for about 5 minutes or until the apples are tender; stir in cinnamon and brown rice and cook for about 5 minutes and then remove from heat.

Serve immediately.

Nutritional Information per Serving:
Calories: 226; Total Fat: 4.3 g; Net Carbs: 34.4 g; Dietary Fiber: 4.8 g; Sugars: 8.6 g; Protein: 5.8 g; Cholesterol: 0 mg; Sodium: 26 mg

10. Buckwheat Cereal with Red Onions & Mushrooms

Yield: 4 Servings
Total Time: 55 Minutes
Prep Time: 15 Minutes
Cook Time: 40 Minutes

Ingredients

- 1 cup buckwheat groats
- 1 tablespoon olive oil, or to taste
- 1 red onion, diced
- 1 carrot, diced
- ½ pound mushrooms, diced
- 1 tablespoon butter
- 2 cups water
- A pinch of sea salt
- A pinch of black pepper

Directions

Rinse buckwheat and drain. Heat a nonstick skillet over medium heat and cook in buckwheat for about 5 minutes or until toasted; transfer to a large bowl and set aside.

Add olive oil to the skillet and cook in onions and carrots for about 10 minutes or until tender; stir in mushrooms and cook for about 5 minutes.

In a pot set over medium heat, melt butter and stir in buckwheat; add in the onion mixture, salt, pepper and water and bring a gentle boil. Simmer for about 20 minutes and then serve right away.

Nutritional Information per Serving:
Calories: 185; Total Fat: 7.5 g; Net Carbs: 22.6 g; Dietary Fiber: 4.5 g; Sugars: 3.7 g Protein: 6 g; Cholesterol: 8 mg; Sodium: 101 mg

11. Superfood Overnight Oats

Yield: 2 Servings
Total Time: 10 Minutes + Chilling Time
Prep Time: 10 Minutes
Cook Time: N/A

Ingredients

- 1/2 cup old-fashioned oats
- 1 teaspoon chia seeds
- 1/2 cup vanilla almond milk (unsweetened)
- 1/4 cup fresh blueberries
- 1/4 banana, chopped
- 1/4 cup chopped fresh pineapple
- 1/4 cup nonfat Greek yogurt
- 1/4 teaspoon cinnamon

Directions

In a small jar, combine oats, chia seeds, almond milk, blueberries, banana, pineapple, yogurt, and cinnamon. Refrigerate overnight.

To serve, remove from the fridge and stir to mix well before serving.

Nutritional Information per Serving:
Calories: 310; Total Fat: 8.4 g; Carbs: 29 g; Dietary Fiber: 5 g; Protein: 10.8 g; Cholesterol: 3 mg; Sodium: 29 mg; Sugars: 10.2 g

12. Low Fat Chilli & Onion Omelet

Yield: 2 Servings
Total Time: 20 Minutes
Prep Time: 10 Minutes
Cook Time: 10 Minutes

Ingredients

- 1 teaspoon olive oil
- 2 red onions, chopped
- 1 green chilli, chopped
- 1 small tomato, chopped
- 2 eggs
- 1 teaspoon lemon juice
- ½ teaspoon turmeric powder
- ½ teaspoon red chilli powder
- 2 tablespoons coriander, chopped
- Salt to taste

Directions

In a bowl, combine chilli, coriander, green chillies, chopped onions and turmeric powder until well blended; whisk in the eggs and season with salt and pepper.

In a skillet, heat oil and then pour in about a third of the mixture; swirl the pan to spread the egg mixture and cook for about 1 minute per side or until the egg is set. Transfer to a plate and keep warm. Repeat with the remaining mixture. Serve hot with chilli sauce and a glass of fresh orange juice or chai for a satisfying breakfast meal.

Nutritional Info per Serving:
Calories: 241; Total Fat: 7.4 g; Carbs: 6.2 g; Dietary Fiber: 1.6 g; Sugars: 3.3 g; Protein: 9.2 g; Cholesterol: 246 mg; Sodium: 174 mg

13. Healthy Buckwheat, Millet and Amaranth Porridge

Yield: 4 servings
Total Time: 40 Minutes
Prep Time: 10 Minutes
Cook Time: 30 Minutes

Ingredients

- 1/2 cup buckwheat groats
- 1/2 cup whole grain amaranth
- 1/2 cup whole grain millet
- 5 cups water
- 1 teaspoon kosher salt
- 1 tablespoon flax seeds
- 2 cups almond milk
- 1 teaspoon ground cinnamon
- 1/8 teaspoon ground nutmeg
- 2 tablespoons raw honey

Directions

Rinse the grains and add to a pot of boiling salted water; lower heat and simmer for about 30 minutes or until the grains are cooked through.

Remove from heat and stir in almond milk; divide among serving bowl and drizzle each serving with raw honey and sprinkle with cinnamon and nutmeg. Enjoy!

Nutritional Info per Serving:
Calories: 318; Total Fat: 3.4 g; Carbs: 55.7 g; Dietary Fiber: 7.3 g; Sugars: 9.3 g; Protein: 9.5 g; Cholesterol: 0 mg; Sodium: 644 mg

14. Ginger Almond Berry Smoothie Bowl

Yield: 2 Servings
Total Time: 10 Minutes
Prep Time: 10 Minutes
Cook Time: N/A

Ingredients

- 1 cup unsweetened almond milk
- 1 scoop vanilla protein powder
- 1 tablespoon ground flaxseed
- 1 cup kale, chopped
- 1 teaspoon minced fresh ginger
- 1 cup frozen, chopped spinach
- 1 cup blueberries
- 1 cup strawberries

Directions

Combine all ingredients in a blender and blend until very smooth and creamy. Divide the smoothie between serving bowls and top each with your favorite toppings. Enjoy!

Nutrition information per Serving:

Calories: 222; Total Fat: 11.2 g; Carbs: 8.1 g; Dietary Fiber: 3.6 g; Sugars: 2.6 g; Protein: 3.7 g; Cholesterol: 0 mg; Sodium: 105 mg

15. Citrus Superfood Breakfast Smoothie Bowl

Yield: 2 Servings
Total Time: 5 Minutes
Prep Time: 5 Minutes
Cook Time: N/A

Ingredients

- 1/2 cup fresh lemon juice
- 1/2 cup fresh orange juice
- 1 cup fresh grapefruit juice
- 1 cup blueberries
- 1 cup baby spinach
- 1 cup chopped kale
- 1/4 avocado
- 2 teaspoons chlorella powder
- 2 teaspoons spirulina powder
- 2 teaspoons matcha powder

Directions

Blend together all ingredients until very smooth. Serve with your favorite toppings.

16. Low Fat Omelets with Mushrooms & Veggies

Yield: 2 Servings
Total Time: 25 Minutes
Prep Time: 10 Minutes
Cook Time: 15 Minutes

Ingredients

- 3 egg whites
- 1 egg
- 1/2 teaspoon extra-virgin olive oil
- 1/8 teaspoon red pepper flakes
- 1/8 teaspoon ground nutmeg
- 1/8 teaspoon garlic powder
- 1/4 teaspoon salt
- 1/8 teaspoon ground black pepper
- 1/2 cup sliced fresh mushrooms
- 2 tablespoons chopped red bell pepper
- 1/4 cup chopped green onion
- 1/2 cup chopped tomato
- 1 cup chopped fresh spinach

Directions

In a large bowl, whisk together egg whites, egg, garlic powder, red pepper flakes, nutmeg, salt and pepper until well blended.

Heat olive oil in a skillet over medium heat; add green onion, mushrooms and belle pepper and cook for about 5 minutes or until tender; stir in tomato and egg mixture and cook for about 5 minutes per side or until egg is set. Slice and serve hot.

Nutrition information per Serving:
Calories: 127; Total Fat: 4 g; Carbs: 13.7 g; Dietary Fiber: 3.1 g; Sugars: 8.4 g; Protein: 11 g; Cholesterol: 82 mg; Sodium: 392 mg

17.Spiced Mushroom Egg Scramble

Yield: 2 Servings
Total Time: 20 Minutes
Prep Time: 10 Minutes
Cook Time: 10 Minutes

Ingredients

- 1 teaspoon coconut oil
- 1 red onion, diced
- 1 Bell Pepper, diced
- 1 cup chopped mushrooms
- 1 teaspoon hot sauce
- 3 free-range eggs
- 1/4 teaspoon red pepper flakes, crushed
- 1/4 teaspoon cumin
- Pinch of sea salt
- Pinch of pepper

Directions

Melt coconut oil in a nonstick skillet set over medium heat; stir in red onions and peppers and sauté for about 4 minutes or until onions are translucent.

Meanwhile, in a bowl, whisk together hot sauce, eggs, crushed red pepper flakes, cumin, salt and pepper until frothy; add to onion mixture and cook, stirring, until eggs are set. Season with salt and pepper and serve with mango chutney.

Nutrition Information per Serving:
Calories: 203; Total Fat: 15.9 g; Carbs: 4.7 g; Dietary Fiber: 1 g; Sugars: 2.7 g Protein: 11.8 g; Cholesterol: 327 mg; Sodium: 528 mg

18. Chai Spiced Greek Yogurt Parfait with Fresh Fruits

Yield: 4 Servings
Total Time: 10 Minutes
Prep Time: 10 Minutes
Cook Time: N/A

Ingredients

- 1 cup granola cereal
- 2 cups non-fat Greek yogurt
- 1/2 teaspoon ground allspice
- 1/2 teaspoon ground ginger
- 1/2 teaspoon ground cardamom
- 1/2 teaspoon ground cloves
- 1/2 teaspoon ground nutmeg
- 1/2 teaspoon ground cinnamon
- 1 banana, sliced
- 1 cup halved apricots

Directions

In a small bowl, stir together yogurt and spices until well combined.

Sprinkle a small layer of granola in a serving glass and then top with a layer of yogurt mixture followed by banana slices and apricot halves; repeat the layers to fill the glasses. Enjoy!

Nutritional Information per Serving:
Calories: 207; Total Fat: 8.4 g; Carbs: 48.6 g; Dietary Fiber: 7.5 g; Sugars: 23.5 g; Protein: 20.2 g; Cholesterol: 9 mg; Sodium: 51 mg

19. Citrus Turmeric Smoothie

Yield: 2 Servings
Total Time: 5 Minutes
Prep Time: 5 Minutes
Cook Time: N/A

Ingredients

- 1 teaspoon turmeric
- ½ an orange, segmented
- 1 cup of Greek yogurt
- ½ cup mango chunks
- ½ cup almond milk
- 1 banana, sliced

Directions

Blend together all ingredients until very smooth. Enjoy!

Nutritional Info per Serving:
Calories: 209; Total Fat: 3.8 g; Carbs: 32.8 g; Dietary Fiber: 3.5 g; Sugars: 24 g; Protein: 13.6 g; Cholesterol: 10 mg; Sodium: 63 mg

20. Mushrooms, Boiled Eggs & Veggie Breakfast Bowl

Yield: 2 Servings
Total Time: 15 Minutes
Prep Time: 5 Minutes
Cook Time: 10 Minutes

Ingredients

- 4 large boiled eggs, diced
- 1 teaspoon extra-virgin olive oil
- 1/2 cup chopped button mushrooms
- 1 cup arugula/baby spinach
- 1/4 cup chopped red onion
- 1/4 cup chopped green bell pepper
- Hot sauce, to serve

Directions

Heat olive oil in a pan set over medium heat; add green bell pepper, onion and mushrooms and sauce for about 5 minutes or until tender.

Stir in arugula and cook for about 5 minutes or until it wilts; add diced boiled eggs and cook for a few minutes.

Serve right away with hot sauce.

Nutrition Information per Serving:

Calories: 201; Total Fat: 6.8 g; Carbs: 4.4 g; Dietary Fiber: 1 g; Sugars: 2.5 g Protein: 13.9 g; Cholesterol: 372 mg; Sodium: 216 mg

21. Spiced Egg Frittata

Yield: 4 Servings
Total Time: 20 Minutes
Prep Time: 10 Minutes
Cook Time: 10 Minutes

Ingredients

- 5 eggs
- 1 teaspoon paprika
- 1 tablespoon curry powder
- ½ teaspoon salt
- ½ teaspoon pepper
- 1 tablespoon chopped cilantro
- 1 cup diced tomatoes
- 2 tablespoons coconut oil
- 1 Serrano pepper, minced
- 1 yellow onion, diced

Directions

Preheat your oven to 350 degrees.

Whisk together eggs, spices and cilantro in a bowl; set aside.
Heat oil in a skillet and then fry in serrano peppers, onions, and salt until onion is soft; add in tomatoes and cook, covered, for 10 minutes or until tomatoes are soft. Add in the egg mixture and stir in to combine. Cook for about 5 minutes and then transfer to the oven. Bake for about minutes or until the egg is set. Serve hot with chai masala.

Nutritional Info per Serving:
Calories: 164; Total Fat: 1.9 g; Carbs: 6.3 g; Dietary Fiber: 2 g; Sugars: 3 g; Protein: 7.9 g; Cholesterol: 205 mg; Sodium: 373 mg

22. Lemon Blueberry Almond Smoothie

Yield: 1 Serving
Total Time: 5 Minutes
Prep Time: 5 Minutes
Cook Time: N/A

Ingredients

- ½ cup fresh lemon juice
- ½ cup almond milk
- 1 cup frozen blueberries
- 1 apple
- 1 pitted date
- 1 piece of fresh ginger root
- ¼ teaspoon ground turmeric
- pinch of pink Himalayan salt

Directions

In a blender, blend together all ingredients until very smooth. Enjoy!

23. The Ultimate Detox Smoothie

Yield: 1 Serving
Total Time: 10 Minutes
Prep Time: 10 Minutes
Cook Time: N/A

Ingredients:

- 1 cup fresh lemon juice
- 2 cups blueberries
- 2 bananas
- 1 tablespoon minced ginger
- 1 teaspoon spirulina
- 1 cup cilantro
- 1 tablespoon chlorella powder

Directions:

Blend together all ingredients in a blender until very smooth. Enjoy!

24. Low Fat Greek Yogurt with Acai Berry Granola

Yield: 2 Servings
Total Time: 5 Minutes
Prep Time: 5 Minutes
Cook time: N/A

Ingredients

- 2 cup nonfat Greek yogurt
- 2 teaspoons raw honey
- ½ cup granola cereal
- ½ cup frozen acai berries

Directions

Pour the yogurt in a serving bowl or a glass and stir in raw honey and top with granola, sprinkle acai berries on top. Enjoy!

Nutritional Information per Serving:

Calories: 230 Total Fat: 18.2 g; Carbs: 45.5 g; Dietary Fiber: 5.5 g; Sugars: 2.2 g; Protein: 29.1 g; Cholesterol: 20mg; Sodium: 120 mg

25. Healthy Millet Porridge

Yield: 2 Servings
Total Time: 40 Minutes
Prep Time: 10 Minutes
Cook Time: 30 Minutes

Ingredients

- 2 cups unsweetened almond milk
- ½ cup hulled millet
- 2 tablespoons slivered almonds
- 2 tablespoons shredded unsweetened coconut
- ¼ teaspoon ground nutmeg
- ½ teaspoon ground cinnamon

Directions

Grind millet in a food processor; set aside.

Toast almonds and walnuts in a nonstick skillet over medium high heat for about 5 minutes or until golden brown. Stir in coconut and almonds and toast for 5 minutes more and then remove from heat.

Add millet to the skillet and toast for about 3 minutes or until fragrant. Stir in 1 ½ cups of almond milk and bring to a gentle boil; lower heat and simmer for about 10 minutes. Stir in the half of the toasted coconut and almonds cinnamon, and nutmeg and simmer for another 10 minutes.

Serve the porridge in two bowls and top with the remaining almond milk and toasted seed mixture.

Nutrition info Per Serving:
Calories: 397; Total Fat: 14.6 g; Net Carbs: 31.7 g; Dietary Fiber: 8.7 g; Sugars: 0.9; Protein: 12.6 g; Cholesterol: 0 mg; Sodium: 186 mg

26. Wholesome Buckwheat Pancakes

Yield: 2 Servings
Total Time: 20 Minutes
Prep Time: 10 Minutes
Cook Time: 10 Minutes

Ingredients

- ⅔ cup raw buckwheat groats, soaked overnight and rinsed
- 1 egg
- ¼ teaspoon cinnamon
- 1 teaspoon stevia
- ¼ teaspoon sea salt
- ½ cup water

Directions

Transfer rinsed and drained buckwheat to a blender and add in egg, stevia, cinnamon, salt and water and blend until very smooth.

Grease a nonstick skillet and set over medium heat; pour in about a third cup of the buckwheat batter, spreading to cover the bottom of the skillet. Cook for about 2 minutes over side of until the pancake is golden brown. Repeat with the remaining batter.
Serve right away with a glass of orange juice.

Nutritional Information per Serving:
Calories: 166; Total Fat: 3.5 g; Net Carbs: 26.4 g; Dietary Fiber: 4.2 g; Sugars: 1.2 g; Protein: 7.8 g; Cholesterol: 82 mg; Sodium: 271 mg

27. Low Fat Sweet Potato & Turkey Breakfast Casserole

Yield: 6 Servings
Total Time: 50 Minutes
Prep Time: 5 Minutes
Cook Time: 45 Minutes

Ingredients

- 1 teaspoon coconut oil
- 1/2-pound ground turkey
- 1 large sweet potato, cut into slices
- 1/2 cup spinach
- 6 eggs
- Salt and pepper

Directions

Preheat oven to 350°F. Lightly coat a square baking tray with coconut oil and set aside. In a skillet set over medium heat, brown ground turkey in coconut oil; season well and remove from heat.

Layer the potato slices onto the baking tray and top with raw spinach and ground turkey. In a small bowl, whisk eggs, salt and pepper until well blended; pour over the mixture to cover completely; bake for about 45 minutes or until eggs are cooked through and the potatoes are tender. Remove from oven and let cool a bit before serving.

Nutrition info Per Serving:
Calories: 247; Total Fat: 5.2 g; Net Carbs: 5.9 g; Dietary Fiber: 1.1 g; Sugars: 2.6; Protein: 22.1 g; Cholesterol: 366 mg; Sodium: 176 mg

LUNCH RECIPES

28. Healthy Millet Lettuce Wraps

Yield: 2 Servings
Total Time: 30 Minutes
Prep Time: 10 Minutes
Cook Time: 20 Minutes

Ingredients

- 4 leaves lettuce
- ¼ cup millet
- 1 teaspoon butter
- ½ cup water
- ¼ red onion, chopped
- 1 clove garlic, minced
- 2 tablespoons fresh lime juice
- 1 teaspoon chopped cilantro
- ½ teaspoon sea salt
- 1 carrot, chopped

Directions

In a skillet, toast millet for about 5 minutes or until fragrant and toasted; transfer to a plate and set aside. Add butter to the skillet and sauté in red onion and garlic for about 3 minutes or until fragrant. Stir in toasted millet, lime juice, cilantro, sea salt and water; simmer for about 10 minutes or until the liquid is absorbed. Remove from heat.
Divide carrots among the lettuce leaves and top each with the millet mixture. Roll to form wraps and serve.

Nutrition info Per Serving:
Calories: 133; Total Fat: 3 g; Net Carbs: 19.9 g; Dietary Fiber: 3.3 g; Sugars: 2.2; Protein: 3.3 g; Cholesterol: 5 mg; Sodium: 507 mg

29. Chickpea Salad Wrap

Yield: 3 Servings
Total Time: 5 Minutes
Prep Time: 5 Minutes
Cook Time: N/A

Ingredients:

- 1 ½ cups cooked chickpeas
- 1/4 cup toasted sunflower seeds
- 1 tablespoon minced fresh dill
- 3 tablespoons chopped dill pickle
- 2 tablespoons chopped red onion
- 1/2 cup chopped celery
- 2 tablespoons fresh lemon juice
- 1/2 tsp regular mustard
- 1 garlic clove, minced
- ¼ teaspoon sea salt
- ¼ teaspoon pepper
- Whole wheat tortillas

Directions:

In a large bowl, mix all the ingredients, mashing the chickpeas until smooth. Stuff the mixture into a wrap and serve.

Nutritional Information per Serving:
Calories: 302 Total Fat: 6.3 g; Carbs: 48.2 g; Dietary Fiber: 14 g; Sugars: 8.8 g; Protein: 15.6 g; Cholesterol: 0 mg; Sodium: 237 mg

30. Warm Bean Soup with Whole-Wheat Tortilla Chips

Yield: 6 Servings
Total Time: 1 Hour 10 Minutes
Prep Time: 10 Minutes
Cook Time: 1 Hour

Ingredients

- 6 cups boiling water
- 1 large red onion, diced
- 1 pound dried black beans
- 1/4 teaspoon chipotle chile powder
- 2 teaspoons cumin
- 1 teaspoon sea salt
- 1 cup salsa
- 12 ounces frozen corn kernels
- 1 tablespoon fresh lime juice
- Avocado slices
- baked Whole-wheat tortilla chips

Directions

Boil water in an instant pot and turn it to sauté setting; add onion and cook, stirring often, until tender and browned.

Stir in beans, chipotle chili powder, cumin, boiling water, and sea salt; turn off the sauté function. Lock lid in place and turn on high pressure, adjusting time to 30 minutes. Let pressure come down naturally before opening the pot.
Remove about 3 cups of beans to a blender and blend until very smooth; return to pot and add salsa and corn. Adjust seasoning and turn the pot on sauté; cook until heated through. Ladle in serving bowls and drizzle with lime juice, garnish with avocado slices and serve with baked tortilla chips.

Nutritional Information per Serving:
Calories: 329; Total Fat: 1 g; Carbs: 65 g; Dietary Fiber: 15 g; Sugars: 7 g; Protein: 18 g; Cholesterol: 0 mg; Sodium: 707 mg

31. Healthy Salad with Hot Berry Dressing

Yield: 4 Servings
Total Time: 5 Minutes
Prep Time: 5 Minutes
Cook Time: N/A

Ingredients

Salad

- 1 cup blueberries
- 1 cup chopped strawberries
- 1 cup chopped kale
- 1 cup arugula
- 1 cup baby spinach
- 2 chopped red onions
- 1 cup shredded carrots
- 1 cup diced tomatoes

Hot Creamy Dressing

- 1 teaspoon extra-virgin olive oil
- 1/4 cup fresh lemon juice
- ¼ cup fresh orange juice
- 1/2 cup fresh berries
- 1 teaspoon raw honey
- 1 teaspoon sea salt
- ½ teaspoon cayenne pepper

Directions

In a blender, blend together all dressing ingredients until very smooth and creamy; set aside. Combine all salad ingredients in a large bowl; drizzle with dressing and toss to coat well before serving.

Nutritional Information per Serving:

Calories: 141; Total Fat: 7.4 g; Carbs: 17.4 g; Dietary Fiber: 5.5 g; Sugars: 7.5 g; Protein: 2.9 g; Cholesterol: 0 mg; Sodium: 42 mg

32. Spiced Sweet Potato and Spring Onion Salad

Yield: 4 Servings
Total Time: 20 Minutes
Prep Time: 10 Minutes
Cook Time: 10 Minutes

Ingredients

- 4 large sweet potatoes, peeled, diced
- 1 cup sliced spring onions
- 1 medium red bell pepper, chopped
- 2 tablespoons minced mint leaves
- 2 fresh minced chillies, chopped
- 1 tablespoon grated orange zest
- 2 teaspoons ground cumin
- ¼ cup apple cider vinegar
- 4 tablespoons extra-virgin olive oil
- ¼ teaspoon sea salt
- ¼ teaspoon black pepper

Directions

Preheat your oven to 350 degrees.

Place sweet potatoes on a baking sheet and drizzle with half of oil; sprinkle with salt and pepper and toss to coat well. Bake in the preheated oven for about 30 minutes or until tender and browned.

Meanwhile, add the remaining oil to the blender along with bell pepper, vinegar, zest, and cumin, sea salt, pepper and blend until very smooth.

Remove the potatoes from the oven and toss with chiles, mint and spring onions. Drizzle with the dressing and toss to coat well. Enjoy!

Nutritional Information per Serving:

Calories: 259; Total Fat: 14.5 g; Net Carbs: 26.2 g; Dietary Fiber: 5.4 g; Sugars: 7.6 g Protein: 3.1 g; Cholesterol: 0 mg; Sodium: 197 mg

33. Low Fat Salad with Ginger & Lemon Dressing

Yield: 2 Servings
Total Time: 10 Minutes
Prep Time: 10 Minutes
Cook Time: N/A

Ingredients

Salad
- 1 cup shredded carrot
- 4 cups shredded purple cabbage
- Handful of fresh chopped cilantro
- 1/2 avocado, sliced
- ½ cup cherry tomatoes
- 2 tablespoons raisins

Ginger Lemon Dressing
- 4 tablespoons freshly squeezed lemon juice
- 2 tablespoons raw honey
- 1 tablespoons chopped fresh ginger
- 1 clove garlic

Directions

In a blender, blend together all dressing ingredients until very smooth; set aside.

In a large bowl, toss together carrots, tomatoes, cabbage, and cilantro and top with raisins and sliced avocado. Drizzle with the dressing and toss to coat well. Let sit for about 10 minutes for the flavors to blend well. Enjoy!

34. Cauliflower & Broccoli Soup

Yield: 4 Servings
Total Time: 25 Minutes
Prep Time: 5 Minutes
Cook Time: 20 Minutes

Ingredients

- 4 cups cauliflower florets
- 8 cups broccoli florets
- 1 teaspoon extra-virgin olive oil
- 1 celery rib, chopped
- 1 small onion, chopped
- 1/8 teaspoon celery seeds
- 1/4 teaspoon white pepper
- 1/2 teaspoon onion powder
- 1/2 teaspoon garlic powder
- 1 teaspoon salt
- 3 cups vegetable broth
- 1 cup almond milk

Directions

In a stock pot, heat olive oil over medium heat and then stir in celery, onion, salt and pepper; cook for about 3 minutes or until fragrant. Stir in celery seeds, garlic powder, onion powder, cauliflower, half of broccoli and vegetable broth. Simmer covered, for about 10 minutes. Transfer the mixture, in batches, to a blender and blend until very smooth; return to the pot. Chop the remaining broccoli and add to the pot along with coconut milk. Simmer for about 3 minutes and then remove from heat to serve.

Nutritional Information per Serving:
Calories: 151; Total Fat: 2.5 g; Carbs: 23 g; Dietary Fiber: 8 g; Sugars: 8g; Protein: 8.1 g; Cholesterol: 0 mg; Sodium: 1457 mg

35. Green Salad with Beets & Edamame

Yield: 2 Servings
Total Time: 15 Minutes
Prep Time: 15 Minutes
Cook Time: N/A

Ingredients

- ½ cup shredded raw beet
- 1 cup shelled edamame, thawed
- 2 cups mixed salad greens
- 1/2 teaspoon extra-virgin olive oil
- 1 tablespoon + 1½ teaspoons apple cider vinegar
- 1 tablespoon chopped fresh cilantro
- Salt & pepper

Directions

In a large bowl, combine beets, edamame and salad greens. In a small bowl, whisk together olive oil, vinegar, cilantro, salt and pepper and drizzle over the salad. Serve chilled.

Nutrition information per Serving:

Calories: 325; Total Fat: 1.6 g; Carbs: 25 g; Dietary Fiber: 12 g; Sugars: 6 g; Protein: 18 g; Cholesterol: 0 mg; Sodium: 499 mg;

36. Winter Savory Soup

Yield: 6 Servings
Total Time: 40 Minutes
Prep Time: 10 Minutes
Cook Time: 30 Minutes

Ingredients
- 225g red lentils
- 100g pearl barley
- 200g sweet potato, cut into chunks
- 200g butternut squash, cut into chunks
- 1 parsnip, cut into chunks
- 2 green chillies, deseeded and finely chopped
- 2 garlic cloves, finely chopped
- 1 large onion, chopped
- 2 tomatoes, chopped
- 1 teaspoon cumin seeds
- ½ teaspoon brown mustard seeds
- 1 teaspoon coconut oil
- 1 teaspoon paprika
- ½ teaspoon ground turmeric
- 1 small cinnamon stick
- 1 teaspoon ground coriander
- 1 teaspoon lemon juice
- 1 teaspoon grated ginger
- small bunch coriander, chopped
- 2 cloves
- 1 bay leaf

Directions
Follow package instructions to cook pearl barley until tender; drain and set aside. In the meantime, heat oil in a pan and fry in cumin seeds, mustard seeds, turmeric, cloves, cinnamon and bay leaf for about 2 minutes or until fragrant; stir in garlic and onion and cook for about 5 minutes. stir in sweet potatoes, butternut and parsnip until well coated with spices. Sprinkle with ground coriander, paprika and seasoning and then add in barley, lentils, tomatoes and water. Bring to a gentle boil and then simmer for about 15 minutes or until the veggies are tender. Stir in lemon juice, ginger and chopped coriander and serve hot.

Nutritional Information per Serving:
Calories: 445; Total Fat: 2.8 g; Carbs: 80 g; Dietary Fiber: 8 g; Sugars: 13 g; Protein: 19 g; Cholesterol: 0mg; Sodium: 140 mg

37. Stir-Fried Mushrooms & Spinach with Golden Onions

Yield: 6 Servings
Total Time: 35 Minutes
Prep Time: 15 Minutes
Cook Time: 20 Minutes

Ingredients

- 1 cup mushrooms, quartered
- 2 medium onions, chop one and thinly slice the other
- 6 cups ready washed young leaf spinach
- 2 teaspoons coconut oil
- 1 small green chilli, chopped
- 1 tablespoon minced ginger
- 1 crushed garlic clove
- ½ teaspoon garlic
- ½ teaspoon garam masala
- ½ teaspoon cumin seeds
- ½ teaspoon turmeric

Directions

Heat two tablespoons of oil in a large pan; fry in cumin seeds for 30 seconds or until fragrant and then add in onion and mushrooms; cook for 10 minutes or until tender. Stir in chilli, ginger, garlic and garam masala. Stir in spinach and cook for 3 minutes or until wilted. Season with salt and serve warm.

In the remaining oil, fry onion slices with turmeric for about 7 minutes or until golden browned. Serve the spinach sprinkled with onions.

Nutritional Information per Serving:
Calories: 103; Total Fat: 3.7 g; Carbs: 5 g; Dietary Fiber: 4 g; Sugars: 0 g; Protein: 5 g; Cholesterol: 11 mg; Sodium: 510 mg

38. Spiced Lentils & Brown Rice Dish

Yield: 3 Servings
Total Time: 5 Minutes
Prep Time: 5 Minutes
Cook Time: N/A

Ingredients

- 5 cups water
- 1 cup mixed lentils and split peas
- 3 tablespoons minced garlic
- 1 teaspoon turmeric
- 1 teaspoon cumin
- 1 teaspoon curry powder
- ½ teaspoon pepper
- ½ teaspoon sea salt
- ½ cup brown rice
- 2 cups frozen veggies

Directions

Bring water to a rolling boil in a pot; add the lentils and split peas, garlic and spices and cook for about 50 minutes or until lentils are tender. Add frozen veggies to lentils and cook for 5 minutes more.

Meanwhile, boil rice in salted water until tender. Serve the lentil-veggie stew over rice.

Nutritional Information per Serving:
Calories: 330 Total Fat: 1.6 g; Carbs: 62 g; Dietary Fiber: 20 g; Sugars: 3.9 g; Protein: 17.4 g; Cholesterol: 0 mg; Sodium: 281 mg

39. Green Bean, Broccoli & Carrot Salad

Yield: 4 Servings
Total Time: 30 Minutes
Prep Time: 15 Minutes
Cook Time: 15 Minutes

Ingredients

- 250g green bean, trimmed
- 1 head of broccoli, cut into florets
- 1 teaspoon olive oil
- 2 tsp black mustard seed
- ½ tsp dried chilli flakes
- 100g pea
- 3 large carrots, grated
- large bunch coriander, roughly chopped

For the dressing

- 200ml nonfat Greek yogurt
- ½ cucumber, peeled and grated
- thumb-sized piece ginger, grated
- ½ tsp ground cumin
- juice and zest 1 lime
- 1 tablespoon chopped mint leaves

Directions

In a pan of boiling salted water, cook green beans for about 3 minutes and then add in broccoli. Cook for 2 minutes and then remove from heat; drain and set aside.

In the meantime, mix together the raita ingredients and set aside.
Add oil to a pa set over medium heat; stir in mustard seeds and chili flakes and sauté for about 5 minutes or until fragrant; stir in the broccoli, green beans and peas and toss until heated through. Remove from heat and stir in coriander and carrots.
Serve the salad warm drizzled with a dollop of the dressing.

Nutritional Information per Serving:
Calories: 248; Total Fat: 4.1 g; Carbs: 21 g; Dietary Fiber: 14 g; Sugars 7 g; Protein: 16 g; Cholesterol: 0 mg; Sodium: 200 mg

40. Spiced Carrot Soup

Yield: 4 Servings
Total Time: 50 Minutes
Prep Time: 10 Minutes
Cook Time: 40 Minutes

Ingredients

- 1 teaspoon olive oil
- 1 cup chopped leek
- 1 cup chopped butternut squash
- 1 cup chopped fennel
- 3 cups chopped carrots
- 1 tablespoon turmeric
- 1 tablespoon grated ginger
- 2 garlic cloves, minced
- 2 cups almond milk
- 3 cups vegetable broth
- Salt & pepper

Directions

Heat oil in a saucepan and then sauté in leeks, fennel, squash, and carrots for about 5 minutes or until tender. Stir in turmeric, ginger, garlic, salt and pepper and cook for about 2 minutes. stir in coconut milk and broth and simmer for about 20 minutes.

Transfer the mixture to a blender and blend until creamy. Serve right away with a dollop of yogurt.

Nutritional Information per Serving:
Calories: 210; Total Fat: 4.9 g; Carbs: 25.6 g; Dietary Fiber: 4.8 g; Sugars: 7.7g; Protein: 2.1 g; Cholesterol: 0 mg; Sodium: 875 mg

41. Spiced Vegetable Indian Soup

Yield: 8 Servings
Total Time: 1 Hour 30 Minutes
Prep Time: 10 Minutes
Cook Time: 1 Hour 20 Minutes

Ingredients

- 4 cups navy beans
- 1 sweet potato, peeled, diced
- 1 clove garlic, minced
- 1 small yellow onion, diced
- 1 stalk celery, diced
- 3 carrots, peeled and sliced
- 1 teaspoon paprika
- 1/8 teaspoon allspice
- 1/2 teaspoon black pepper
- ¼ teaspoon sea salt
- 2 cups diced tomatoes
- 4 cups vegetable broth
- 1 bay leaf
- 4 cups baby spinach
- 1 teaspoon extra-virgin olive oil

Directions

Combine all ingredients, except olive oil and spinach, in a slow cooker. Cook, covered, for about 7 hours or until the veggies are tender; remove the pot from heat and mash the ingredients with a fork. Return to the pot and continue cooking for 1 hour more. Stir in spinach and cook, for about 5 minutes or until wilted. Serve drizzled with a splash of extra virgin olive oil. Enjoy!

Nutritional Information per Serving:
Calories: 253; Total Fat: 4 g; Carbs: 43 g; Dietary Fiber: 9 g; Protein: 12 g; Cholesterol: 1 mg; Sodium: 75 mg; Sugars: 6 g

42. Spiced Healthy Cauliflower Bowl

Yield: 8 Servings
Total Time: 30 Minutes
Prep Time: 10 Minutes
Cook Time: 20 Minutes

Ingredients

- 1¼kg cauliflower, broken into pieces
- 1 tablespoon chopped ginger
- 2 red onions, chopped
- 4 cloves garlic, minced
- 1 teaspoon vegetable oil
- 2 teaspoon turmeric
- 2 tablespoons cumin seed
- 2 teaspoons chilli flakes
- 1 tablespoon chopped coriander

Directions

Heat oil in a wok and stir in onions, garlic, and ginger and all the spices for about 40 seconds or until fragrant; lower heat and stir in cauliflower and seasoning. Cook, covered, for 10 minutes or until tender and then remove from heat. Serve in a bowl garnished with coriander.

Nutritional Information per Serving:
Calories: 145; Total Fat: 10 g; Carbs: 7 g; Dietary Fiber: 3 g; Sugars: 4 g; Protein: 6 g; Cholesterol: 3 mg; Sodium: 50 mg

43. Raw Vegetable & Papaya Salad

Yield: 2 Servings
Total Time: 10 Minutes
Prep Time: 10 Minutes
Cook Time: N/A

Ingredients

- 1 cup grated carrots
- 1 cup shredded purple cabbage
- 2 cup chopped lettuce
- 1 cup diced papaya
- 2 tablespoons fresh lemon juice
- 2 tablespoons extra-virgin olive oil
- 1 tablespoon apple cider vinegar

Directions

Mix all salad ingredients until well combined; drizzle with fresh lemon juice, apple cider vinegar, and extra virgin olive oil and toss to coat well/ season with salt and pepper and serve.

44. Superfood Nutty Salad with Hot Citrus Dressing

Yield: 6 Servings
Total Time: 10 Minutes
Prep Time: 10 Minutes
Cook Time: N/A

Salad:
- 1 cup shredded red cabbage
- 1 cup chopped broccoli florets
- 1 cup chopped Brussels sprouts
- 1 cup chopped kale
- 1 cup chopped carrots
- 11 avocado, sliced
- 1/2 cup chopped cilantro
- 1 tablespoon raisins
- 2 tablespoons toasted pumpkin seeds
- 2 tablespoons toasted sunflower seeds

Dressing:
- 1 teaspoon extra-virgin olive oil
- ¼ cup lemon juice
- ¼ cup lime juice
- ¼ cup orange juice
- 2 teaspoons minced fresh jalapeno pepper
- 1 teaspoon minced hot pepper
- ¼ cup snipped fresh cilantro
- ¼ teaspoon salt
- ⅛ teaspoon ground black pepper

Directions

In a jar, combine together all the dressing ingredients until well blended. Set aside.
In a bowl, mix all the salad ingredients; pour in the dressing and toss to coat well. Enjoy!

45. Detox Lemon Leek & Broccoli Soup

Yield: 3 Servings
Total Time: 40 Minutes
Prep Time: 20 Minutes
Cook Time: 20 Minutes

Ingredients

- 1 teaspoon extra-virgin olive oil
- 1 cup chopped leek
- 1 cup chopped red onions
- 1/2 cup chopped celery
- 2 garlic cloves, crushed
- 2 teaspoons grated lemon rind
- 2 potatoes, chopped
- 2 cup homemade vegetable stock
- 1 large zucchini, chopped
- 2 cups chopped broccoli
- 1 cup baby spinach
- 2 tablespoons coconut cream
- Chopped cilantro

Directions

In a skillet, heat oil and sauté red onions, leeks and celery for about 5 minutes or until fragrant and tender; stir in lemon rind and garlic and cook for 1 minute. Add in stock and potatoes and bring the mixture to a boil. Lower the heat and simmer for about 5 minutes. stir in broccoli and zucchini and cook for about 10 minutes. stir in spinach for about 3 minutes or until wilted.

Remove from heat and let cool. Transfer the soup to the food processor and blend until smooth. Return to the pan and cook for about 5 minutes or until warmed through. Serve topped with cilantro.

46. Low Fat Lemon & Turmeric Lentil Soup

Yield: 4 Servings
Total Time: 1 Hour
Prep Time: 15 Minutes
Cook Time: 45 Minutes

Ingredients
- 1 teaspoon extra virgin olive oil
- 1 cup chopped red onion
- 1 cup chopped celery
- 2 teaspoons grated lemon rind
- 2 garlic cloves, crushed
- 1/2 teaspoon dried chili flakes
- 1/2 teaspoon ground cinnamon
- 1 teaspoon turmeric powder
- 2 tomatoes, chopped
- 3/4 cup green lentils, cooked
- 1 cup chopped kale
- 1 cup sliced green beans
- 3 cups homemade vegetable stock
- 4 tablespoons fresh lemon juice
- 2 tablespoons chopped fresh coriander

Directions

Heat olive oil in a skillet set over medium heat; sauté onions and celery for about 5 minutes or until tender. Stir in lemon rind, garlic, chili flakes, cinnamon, and turmeric for about 1 minute or until fragrant.

Stir in lentils, tomatoes, and stock and bring the mixture to a gentle boil. Lower heat and simmer for about 30 minutes or until the lentils are tender. Stir in kale and green beans and cook for 3 minutes. Stir in salt, pepper, coriander and lemon juice and remove the skillet from heat. Blend and serve right away.

47. Vitamin-Rich Salad

Yield: 2 Servings
Total Time: 5 Minutes
Prep Time: 5 Minutes
Cook Time: N/A

Ingredients

- 1 apple, diced
- 2 medium carrots, grated
- 1 red beet, grated
- 1 stem green onion, chopped

Dressing:

- 2 tablespoons apple cider vinegar
- 1/4 fresh lemon juice
- 1 teaspoon extra-virgin olive oil
- 1 tablespoon raw honey
- 1 teaspoon sea salt
- ¼ teaspoon cayenne pepper

Directions

In a bowl, combine diced apple, carrots, beet, and green onions until well combined.

In a small bowl, combine vinegar, lemon juice, olive oil, raw honey, sea salt and cayenne pepper until well blended; pour over the salad and toss until well coated.

Serve right away.

Nutritional Information Per Serving:

Calories: 225; Total Fat: 3.9 g; Carbs: 29.1 g; Dietary Fiber: 8.2 g; Sugars: 18.4 g; Protein: 16.3 g; Cholesterol: 0 mg; Sodium: 50 mg

48. Stir-Fried Beef, Shiitake Mushrooms and Peppers

Yield: 4 Servings
Total Time: 20 Minutes
Prep Time: 10 Minutes
Cook Time: 10 Minutes

Ingredients:

- 1 pound grass-fed lean steak, thinly sliced strips
- 4 cups diced shiitake mushrooms
- 2 tablespoons fresh lemon juice
- 2 teaspoons apple cider vinegar
- Pinch of sea salt
- pinch of pepper
- 1 teaspoon extra-virgin olive oil
- 1 large yellow onion, thinly chopped
- 1/2 red bell pepper, thinly sliced
- 1/2 green bell pepper, thinly sliced
- 1 teaspoon crushed red pepper flakes

Directions:

Place meat in a bowl; stir in lemon juice, apple cider vinegar, sea salt and pepper. Toss to coat well.

Heat a tablespoon of olive oil in a pan set over medium high heat; add meat and cook for about 1 minute or until meat is browned; stir for another 2 minutes and then remove from heat. Heat the remaining oil to the pan and sauté onions for about 2 minutes or until caramelized; stir in mushrooms for about 5 minutes and then stir in peppers; cook for 2 minutes more and return meat to pan and stir in red pepper flakes. Serve hot!

Nutritional Information per Serving:

Calories: 296; Total Fat: 4.3 g; Carbs: 8.3 g; Dietary Fiber: 1.6 g; Sugars: 4.2 g; Protein: 32.76 g; Cholesterol: 62 mg; Sodium: 157 mg

49. Low Fat Vegetable & Orange Salad with Citrus Ginger Dressing

Yield: 8 Servings
Total Time: 10 Minutes
Prep Time: 10 Minutes
Cook Time: N/A

Ingredients

For the dressing
- 2 teaspoons cup olive oil
- 2 teaspoons raw honey
- 3 tablespoons fresh lemon juice
- 2 tablespoons orange juice
- ½ teaspoon finely grated orange zest
- 1 teaspoon Dijon mustard
- 1 garlic clove, crushed
- 2 teaspoons freshly grated ginger

For the salad
- 1 cup watercress, large stalks removed and chopped
- 1 cup lamb's lettuce, chopped
- 1/2 cup chopped chicory
- 3 oranges, peeled, segmented, and deseeded

Directions

In a jar, combine all dressing ingredients and shake to mix well. Chill in the refrigerator for at least 2 days before using.

Combine all salad ingredients and chill for at least 1 hour. When ready, drizzle with dressing and mix to coat well. Enjoy!

Nutritional Information per Serving:
Calories: 143; Total Fat: 4.2 g; Carbs: 8 g; Dietary Fiber: 2 g; Sugars: 1 g; Protein: 2 g; Cholesterol: 0 mg; Sodium: 70 mg

DINNER RECIPES

50. Beef & Sweet Potato Enchilada Casserole

Yield: 10 Servings
Total Time: 40 Minutes
Prep Time: 20 Minutes
Cook Time: 20 Minutes

Ingredients

- 2 sweet potatoes
- 1 pound ground beef
- 1 can black beans, drained
- 1 cup frozen corn
- 1 can red enchilada sauce
- 4 tablespoon chopped fresh cilantro
- 2 teaspoon ground cumin
- 1 teaspoon garlic powder
- 1 teaspoon onion powder
- 12 corn tortillas
- 1 small can diced olives
- 4 tablespoons coconut cream

Directions

Peel and cook the sweet potatoes; mash and mix with 2 tablespoons of cilantro.

Cook the ground beef and then stir in beans, corn, sauce and spices until well combined. Layer half of the meat mixture in a 9x13-inch pan and top with half of corn tortilla; sprinkle with half of the coconut cream and repeat the layers. Top with sweet potatoes, olives and cilantro. Cover with the remaining cream and bake at 350°F for about 25 minutes or until cheese is melted.

Nutritional information per serving:
Calories: 315; Total Fat: 8.2 g; Net Carbs: 5.4 g; Dietary Fiber: 12.5 g; Sugars: 3.2 g; Protein: 31.6 g; Cholesterol: 54 mg; Sodium: 172 mg

51. Delicious Buckwheat with Mushrooms & Green Onions

Yield: 6 Servings
Total Time: 55 Minutes
Prep Time: 20 Minutes
Cook Time: 35 Minutes

Ingredients

- 1 cup uncooked buckwheat
- 2 cup water
- 2 cups mushrooms
- 1 red onion, chopped
- 1 cup chopped green onions
- 3 tablespoons butter
- A pinch of salt and pepper

Directions

Combine buckwheat, salt, and water in a pan   bring to a boil; cook for 25 minutes or until liquid is absorbed.

Melt butter in a pan and fry in red onion until tender; stir in mushrooms and cook for about 5 minutes or until golden brown. Stir in cooked buckwheat and remove from heat. Serve topped with freshly chopped green onions.

Nutrition info Per Serving:

Calories: 166; Total Fat: 6.8 g; Net Carbs: 20.1 g; Dietary Fiber: 3.9 g; Sugars: 1.6; Protein: 5.1 g; Cholesterol: 15 mg; Sodium: 48 mg

52. Yummy Chicken and Sweet Potato Stew

Yield: 4-6 Servings
Total Time: 4-8 Hours
Prep Time: 15 Minutes
Cook Time: 4-8 Hours

Ingredients

- 1-pound boneless chicken breasts, with skin removed and cut into chunks
- 1 Vidalia onion, chopped
- 4 cloves garlic, crushed
- 3 carrots, peeled and diced
- 1 sweet potato, peeled and cut into cubes
- 2 cups chicken broth, preferably homemade
- 3 tablespoons balsamic vinegar
- 2-4 tablespoons tomato paste
- 2 teaspoons whole grain mustard
- 2 cups fresh baby spinach
- Freshly ground pepper and salt to taste

Directions

Combine all the ingredients in your slow cooker and stir well until evenly combined.

Cover and cook on low for 6 to 8 hours or on high for 4-5 hours.
When left with a few minutes of cook time, stir in the baby spinach.
Serve hot.

Nutritional Information per Serving:
Calories: 139 Total Fat: 3.7g; Net Carbs: 2.6 g; Dietary Fiber: 3.8 g; Sugars: 1.2 g; Protein: 5.4 g Sodium: 224mg; sugars: 5.8g

53. Healthy Black Bean Chili

Yield: 4-6 Servings
Total Time: 1 Hour 55 Minutes
Prep Time: 20 Minutes
Cook Time: 1 hour 35 Minutes

Ingredients

- 1 teaspoon extra-virgin olive oil
- 1 red onion, finely chopped
- 3 cloves garlic, finely chopped
- 2 stalks celery, chopped
- 1 green bell pepper, chopped
- 2 red bell peppers, chopped
- 1 ½ cups chopped tomatoes
- Pinch of salt and pepper
- 1 ½ cups black beans
- 1 tablespoon cumin powder
- 2 teaspoons cinnamon powder
- 1 fresh red chili, deseeded and finely chopped
- 1 cup almond milk
- 1 bunch fresh coriander, finely chopped
- Brown rice, to serve

Directions

Heat extra virgin olive oil in a skillet set over medium heat until hot, but not smoky; stir in red onion, garlic and celery until fragrant.

Stir in bell peppers and tomatoes and season with salt and pepper; cook for about 2 minutes and then stir in the black beans. Cook for about 5 minutes and then stir in the spices and almond milk. Simmer for a few minutes or until thick.
Serve over a bed of steamed brown rice sprinkled with coriander and with sliced avocado on the side, if desired.

Nutritional Information per Serving:
Calories: 358; Total Fat: 8.6 g; Net Carbs: 43.5 g; Dietary Fiber: 13.4g; Sugars: 6.2 g; Protein: 12.4 g; Cholesterol: 16 mg; Sodium: 30 mg

54. Healthy Fried Brown Rice with Peas & Prawns

Yield: 8 Servings
Total Time: 20 Minutes
Prep Time: 10 Minutes
Cook Time: 10 Minutes

Ingredients
- 1/2 cup frozen pea
- 2 cups cooked brown rice
- 2 teaspoons extra-virgin olive oil
- 1 red chilli, sliced
- 2 garlic cloves, sliced
- 1 red onion, sliced
- 1 cup large peeled prawn
- 1 bunch coriander, chopped
- 1 tablespoon fish sauce
- 1 tablespoon dark soy sauce
- 4 large eggs
- 1 tablespoon chilli sauce

Directions

Sauté garlic, onion and chilli in hot oil in a skillet for about 3 minutes or until golden; stir in prawns for about 1 minute and then toss in peas and rice. Cook until heated through. Stir in fish sauce, soy sauce and coriander and cook for a minute.

Remove from heat and keep warm. Heat oil in a pan and fry the eggs; season.

Divide rice mixture among four serving plates and top each with a fried egg. Serve with chili sauce topped with coriander.

Nutritional Info per Serving:
Calories: 278; Total Fat: 4.3 g; Carbs: 44.9 g; Dietary Fiber: 3 g; Sugars: 5.4 g; Protein: 8.3 g; Cholesterol: 95 mg; Sodium: 1096 mg

55. Asparagus Quinoa & Steak Bowl

Yield: 4 Servings
Total Time: 25 Minutes
Prep Time: 10
Cook Time: 15 Minutes

Ingredients

- 1-1/2 cups white quinoa
- Olive oil cooking spray
- 3/4 pound lean steak, diced
- 1/2 tsp. low-sodium steak seasoning
- 1/2 cup chopped red bell pepper
- 1/2 cup chopped red onion
- 1 cup frozen asparagus cuts
- 2 ½ tbsp. soy sauce

Directions

Follow package instructions to cook quinoa.

In the meantime, coat a large skillet with cooking spray and heat over medium high heat. Sprinkle beef with the steak seasoning and cook in the skillet for about 3 minutes; add bell pepper and red onion and cook for 3 minutes more or until beef is browned. Add asparagus and continue cooking for 4 minutes or until asparagus is heated through.
Stir soy sauce to the quinoa until well combined and toss it with the beef mixture before serving.

Nutritional Info per Serving:
Calories: 325; Total Fat: 8.2 g; Carbs: 17.4 g; Dietary Fiber: 11.1 g; Sugars: 6.2 g; Protein: 26.3 g; Cholesterol: 121 mg; Sodium: 984 mg

56. Seared Lemon Steak with Vegetables Stir-Fry

Yield: 3- 4 Servings
Total Time: 25 Minutes
Prep Time: 15 Minutes
Cook Time: 10 Minutes

Ingredients for

- 1 pound lean steak
- ¼ cup fresh lemon juice
- 1 tablespoon lemon zest
- 1 ½ cups almond milk
- 2 teaspoons coconut oil
- 1 cup chopped red onion
- 4 cloves garlic, minced
- 2 cups shiitake mushrooms, diced
- 3 medium zucchinis
- 1 green pepper bell
- 1 red pepper bell
- 3 tomatoes
- 1 teaspoon curry powder
- 1 tablespoon ginger
- ¼ teaspoon salt
- ¼ teaspoon pepper

Directions

Rub the meat with lemon juice and sprinkle salt, lemon zest, and cayenne pepper; heat half of coconut oil in a skillet set over medium heat and sear in the meat for about 6 minutes per side or until cooked through and golden browned on the outside. Keep the meat warm wrapped in a foil. Dice zucchinis, bell peppers, tomatoes, and beans in bite-size pieces. Heat oil in a pan and fry the red onion and garlic; add in mushrooms, zucchini, and bell peppers; fry for 3 minutes more. Stir in almond milk and tomatoes and cook for a few minutes. Season with ginger, curry powder, salt and pepper. Serve topped with sliced steak.

Nutritional Information Per Serving:

Calories: 406; Total Fat: 33.6 g; Carbs: 20.2 g; Dietary Fiber: 8 g; Sugars: 9.5 g; Protein: 15.1 g; Cholesterol: 0 mg; Sodium: 50 mg

57. Vegetable Tabbouleh

Yield: 2 Servings
Total Time: 15 Minutes
Prep Time: 5 Minutes
Cook Time: 10 Minutes

Ingredients

- 1 cup broccoli florets
- 1 chopped carrots
- 1 cup shredded cabbage
- 1 teaspoon sesame seeds
- A pinch of salt and pepper
- 1 cup cooked quinoa
- 1 cucumber, sliced
- ¼ cup fresh lemon juice
- Handful cilantro

Directions

Heat oil in a skillet set over medium heat until hot, but not smoky; stir-fry in red onions, garlic, broccoli florets, chopped fresh chili, chopped carrots, shredded cabbage, and sesame seeds. Cook for about 5 minutes or until the veggies are crisp tender. Season with salt and pepper and remove from heat.

Serve with cooked quinoa topped with cucumber and chopped cilantro; drizzle with fresh lemon juice for a healthy flavorful meal.

58. Peppered Steak with Cherry Tomatoes

Yield: 4 Servings
Total Time: 25 Minutes
Prep Time: 10 Minutes
Cook Time: 10 Minutes

Ingredients

- 4 (250g) lean beef steaks
- 1 tablespoon extra-virgin olive oil
- 2 tablespoons pepper
- 1 bunch rocket
- 2 cups cherry tomatoes
- 4 cups green salad
- olive oil cooking spray

Directions

Brush the steak with oil. Place the pepper on a large plate and press the steaks into the pepper until well coated.

Pre heat your chargrill or barbecue grill on medium high and barbecue the steaks for about 5 minutes per side or until cooked well.
Transfer the cooed steaks to a plate and keep warm.
In the meantime, sprat the tomatoes with oil and barbecue them, turning occasionally, for about 5 minutes or until tender.
Arrange the rocket on serving plates and add steaks and tomatoes; serve with green salad.

Nutritional Info per Serving:
Calories: 237; Total Fat: 11.1g; Carbs: 10.7g; Dietary Fiber: 8.1g; Sugars: 2.1g; Protein: 14.8g; Cholesterol: 45mg; Sodium: 35mg

59. Grilled Chicken Breast with Non-Fat Yogurt

Yield: 3 Servings
Total Time: 2 Hours 10 Minutes
Prep Time: 2 Hours
Cook Time: 10 Minutes

Ingredients

For the Grilled Chicken:

- 3 boneless chicken breast halves, skinned
- 1 clove garlic, minced
- 1 tablespoon lemon juice, freshly squeezed
- 1 teaspoon extra virgin olive oil
- 1 teaspoon dried oregano
- Salt and freshly ground black pepper, to taste

For the yogurt:

- 1 cup nonfat Greek yogurt
- 1 clove garlic, minced
- 1 tsp. fresh dill, minced
- ½ cup cucumber, very thinly sliced or shredded

Directions

Use a sharp knife to gently slice through the thickest part of the chicken breast with cutting all the way through so you are able to open it up like a book. Do this for the other two halves. Marinate the chicken with the remaining chicken ingredients in a large bowl. Cover with cling wrap and set in the fridge for 1 ½ to 2 hours. Preheat your grill to medium-high heat. Take out the chicken from the marinade. Lightly grease your grill rack then place the breasts on top. Cook for about 3 minutes on each side or until done to desire. Meanwhile, combine all the yogurt ingredients in a medium bowl.

To serve, serve each breast on a large plate. Place a dollop of the nutty yogurt on the side.

Enjoy!

Nutritional Information per Serving:

Calories: 318; Total Fat: 33. g; Carbs: 8 g; Dietary Fiber: 4 g; Protein: 37.2 g; Cholesterol: 38 mg; Sodium: 468 mg

60. Delicious Low Fat Chicken Curry

Yield: 1 Serving
Total Time: 30 Minutes
Prep Time: 10 Minutes
Cook Time: 20 Minutes

Ingredients

- 100 grams chicken, diced
- ¼ cup chicken broth
- Pinch of turmeric
- Dash of onion powder
- 1 tablespoon minced red onion
- Pinch of garlic powder
- ¼ teaspoon curry powder
- Pinch of sea salt
- Pinch of pepper
- Stevia, optional
- Pinch of cayenne

Directions

In a small saucepan, stir spices in chicken broth until dissolved; stir in chicken, garlic, onion, and stevia and cook until chicken is cooked through and liquid is reduced by half. Serve hot.

Nutritional Information per Serving:

Calories: 170; Total Fat: 3.5 g; Carbs: 2.3 g; Dietary Fiber: 0.6 g; Sugars: 0.8 g; Protein: 30.5 g; Cholesterol: 77 mg; Sodium: 255 mg

61. Tilapia with Mushroom Sauce

Yields: 4 Servings
Total Time: 35 Minutes
Prep Time: 15 Minutes
Cook Time: 20 Minutes

Ingredients

- 4 ounces tilapia fillets
- 2 teaspoon arrow root
- 1 cup mushrooms, sliced
- 1 clove garlic, finely chopped
- 1 small onion, thinly sliced
- 1 teaspoon extra-virgin olive oil
- ½ cup fresh parsley, roughly chopped
- 1 teaspoon thyme leaves, finely chopped
- ½ cup water
- A pinch of freshly ground black pepper
- A pinch of sea salt

Directions

Preheat your oven to 350°F.

Add extra virgin olive oil to a frying pan set over medium heat; sauté onion, garlic and mushrooms for about 4 minutes or until mushrooms are slightly tender.
Stir in arrowroot, sea salt, thyme and pepper and cook for about 1 minute.
Stir in water until thickened; stir in parsley and cook for 1 minute more.
Place the fillets on a baking tray lined with parchment paper; cover the fish with mushroom sauce and bake for about 20 minutes or until the fish is cooked through.

Nutritional Information per Serving:
Calories: 177; Total Fat: 3.7 g; Carbs: 3.3 g; Dietary Fiber: 1.4 g; Sugars: 1.1 g; Protein: 14.9 g; Cholesterol: 1 mg; Sodium: 66 mg

62. Ginger Chicken with Veggies

Yields: 4 Servings
Total Time: 15 Minutes
Prep Time: 10 Minutes
Cook Time: 5 Minutes

Ingredients

- 2 cup skinless, boneless, and cooked chicken breast meat, diced
- 1 teaspoon extra virgin olive
- 1 teaspoon powdered ginger
- 2 red onions, sliced
- 4 cloves garlic, minced
- 1 bell pepper, sliced
- 1 cup thinly sliced carrots
- 1 cup finely chopped celery
- 1 cup chicken broth (not salted)

Directions

Add the oil to a skillet set over medium heat; sauté onion and garlic until translucent. Stir in the remaining ingredients and simmer for a few minutes or until the veggies are tender.

Nutritional Info Per Serving:

Calories: 425; Fat: 21.1g; Carbs: 6.5 g; Dietary Fiber: 3.2 g; Sugars: 1.1 g; Protein: 52g; Cholesterol: 107 mg; Sodium: 110 mg

63. Hot Lemon Prawns

Yield: 4 Servings
Total Time: 27 Minutes
Prep Time: 15 Minutes
Cook Time: 12 Minutes

Ingredients

- 400g raw king prawns
- 1 teaspoon coconut oil
- 40g ginger, grated
- 2-4 green chillies, halved
- 4 curry leaves
- 1 onion, sliced
- 4 teaspoons lemon juice
- 3-4 teaspoons red chilli powder
- 2 teaspoons turmeric
- 1 teaspoon black pepper
- 40g grated coconut
- ½ small bunch coriander

Directions

Rinse the prawns and pat dry with a kitchen towel; add them to a large bowl and then toss in chili powder, turmeric, grated ginger, and lemon juice; set aside.

Heat oil in a saucepan and sauté onion, ginger, chilli, and curry leaves for about 10 minutes or until translucent. Stir in black pepper and then add in prawns along with the marinade. Cook for about 2 minutes or until cooked through. Season and drizzle with extra lemon juice. Serve the prawns sprinkled with coriander and grated coconut. Enjoy!

Nutritional Information per Serving:
Calories: 171; Total Fat: 8 g; Carbs: 4 g; Dietary Fiber: 3 g; Sugars: 1 g; Protein: 19 g; Cholesterol: 0 mg; Sodium: 802 mg

64. Delicious Chicken Tikka Skewers

Yield: 4 Servings
Total Time: 40 Minutes
Prep Time: 20 Minutes
Cook Time: 20 Minutes

Ingredients

- 4 boneless, skinless chicken breasts, diced
- 2 tablespoons hot curry paste
- 1 red onion, sliced
- ½ cucumber, sliced
- For the cucumber salad
- 250g pack cherry tomatoes
- 50g pack lamb's lettuce
- juice 1 lemon
- 150g nonfat Greek yogurt
- handful chopped coriander leaves

Directions

Soak skewers in a bowl of water.

In a bowl, mix together curry paste and yogurt; add in chicken and then marinate for 1 hour.
Meanwhile, toss together red onion, cucumber, coriander, and fresh lemon juice in a bowl. Refrigerate until ready to serve.
Thread chicken and cherry tomatoes on the skewers and grill for about 20 minutes or until cooked through and golden browned on the outside.
Add the lettuce into the salad and stir in mix well; divide among serving bowls and top each with two chicken skewers. Enjoy!

Nutritional Information per Serving:
Calories: 234; Total Fat: 4 g; Carbs: 9.7 g; Dietary Fiber: 2.7 g; Sugars: 8.3g; Protein: 40 g; Cholesterol: 394 mg; Sodium: 773 mg

65. Grilled Chicken with Salad Wrap

Yield: 2 Servings
Total Time: 10 Minutes
Prep Time: 10 Minutes
Cook Time: N/A

Ingredients

- 2 lettuce leaves
- ½ coddled egg
- 1 cup diced cherry tomatoes
- 6 cups chopped curly kale
- 8 ounces sliced grilled chicken
- 1 clove garlic, minced
- 1/2 teaspoon Dijon mustard
- 1 teaspoon raw honey
- 1 teaspoon olive oil
- 1/8 cup fresh lemon juice
- Salt & pepper

Directions

In a large bowl, whisk together half of the egg, honey, mustard, minced garlic, olive oil, fresh lemon juice, salt and pepper until well combined.

Add in cherry tomatoes, chicken and kale and toss to coat well; spread the mixture onto lettuce leaves and roll to form wraps. Slice in half and serve right away!

Nutritional Information per Serving:
Calories: 386; Total Fat: 2.6 g; Carbs: 28.5 g; Dietary Fiber: 4.3 g; Sugars: 5.7 g; Protein: 32.5 g; Cholesterol: 114 mg; Sodium: 183 mg

66. Authentic and Easy Shrimp Curry

Yield: 4 Servings
Total Time: 25 Minutes
Prep Time: 10 Minutes
Cook Time: 15 Minutes

Ingredients

- 1 1/2 pounds medium shrimp, deveined
- 1 teaspoon olive oil
- 1 large onion, chopped
- 1 teaspoon ground red chile pepper
- 1 tablespoon ginger garlic paste
- 1 tomato, finely chopped
- 1 teaspoon ground coriander
- 1/2 teaspoon ground turmeric
- 10 fresh curry leaves
- 1 teaspoon garam masala
- chopped fresh cilantro
- 1/4 cup water
- 2/3 teaspoon salt

Directions

Heat oil in a large saucepan and then sauté onions for about 5 minutes or until fragrant and lightly browned; stir in ginger, cilantro, curry leaves, garlic paste, and salt. Cook for 1 minute.

Mix in shrimp, tomato, turmeric, chile powder and water; lower heat and cook for 8 minutes or until shrimp is no longer pink. Season with garam masala and then remove from heat. Serve over rice or flat bread, garnished with cilantro. Enjoy!

Nutritional Information per Serving:
Calories: 270; Total Fat: 4.8 g; Carbs: 5.3 g; Dietary Fiber: 2.8 g; Sugars: 2.7 g; Protein: 30.7 g; Cholesterol: 277 mg; Sodium: 734 mg

67. Spiced Almond Milk Lentil Stew

Yield: 4 Servings
Total Time: 8 hours 45 Minutes
Prep Time: 15 Minutes
Cook Time: 8 Hours 30 Minutes

Ingredients

- 1 cup dry red lentils, rinsed
- 2 red onions, finely chopped
- 3 cloves garlic, minced
- 1 tbsp. ginger, peeled and minced
- 400g can chopped tomatoes
- 1 cup almond milk
- 2 cups vegetable broth
- 1 teaspoon coconut oil
- 1 teaspoon cumin seed
- 1 teaspoon ground coriander
- 1 teaspoon freshly ground black pepper
- Salt and chili flakes to taste

Directions

Pour the oil into a skillet over medium heat. Sauté the onions for 3 minutes then stir in the ginger, garlic, cumin, coriander and black pepper. Keep stirring for a minute or so then stir in the tomatoes, lentils and stock.

Transfer to your slow cooker and cook on low for 8 hours.
Slowly add the coconut milk and season with salt and chili flakes. Cook for an additional 30 minutes then turn off the slow cooker.
Let the lentil stew cool completely before transferring it into freezer bags or jars.

Nutritional Information per Serving:
Calories: 409; Total Fat: 3.5 g; Carbs: 43.9 g; Dietary Fiber: 18.8 g; Sugars: 8.4 g; Protein: 18.1 g; Cholesterol: 0 mg; Sodium: 403 mg

SNACKS/DESSERTS

68. Healthy Taro Chips

Yield: 4 Servings
Total Time: 30 Minutes
Prep Time: 10 Minutes
Cook Time: 20 Minutes

Ingredients

- 1 pound taro peeled
- 1 teaspoon olive oil
- A pinch of salt
- A pinch of pepper

Directions

With a mandolin, slice the taro lengthwise; place the taro slices on a paper-lined baking sheets and brush with olive oil. Sprinkle with sea salt and pepper and bake at 400 degrees for about 20 minutes or until crisp.

Nutritional Information per Serving:

Calories: 137 Total Fat: 1.4 g; Net Carbs: 25.3 g; Dietary Fiber: 4.7 g; Sugars: 0.5 g; Protein: 1.7 g; Cholesterol: 0 mg; Sodium: 51 mg

69. Amaranth Pop Corns

Yield: 2 Servings
Total Time: 15 Minutes
Prep Time: 5 Minutes
Cook Time: 10 Minutes

Ingredients

- 1/2 cup amaranth seeds
- 1 teaspoon olive oil
- 1 teaspoon cinnamon
- ½ teaspoon sea salt

Directions

Heat olive oil in a pot set over high heat; add in the amaranth seeds and cook until they start popping. Cover the pot and let all seeds pops.

Serve sprinkled with cinnamon and sea salt.

Nutritional Information per Serving:
Calories: 205 Total Fat: 5.5 g; Net Carbs: 28.1 g; Dietary Fiber: 5.1 g; Sugars: 0.8 g; Protein: 7.1 g; Cholesterol: 0 mg; Sodium: 478 mg

70. Beef & Millet Stuffed Peppers

Yield: 4 Servings
Total Time: Hour 20 Minutes
Prep Time: 20 Minutes
Cook Time: 1 Hour

Ingredients
- 4 red bell peppers, tops removed
- ½ cup millet
- ½ pound ground beef
- 2 tablespoons olive oil
- 2 cups water
- 1 onion, chopped
- 2 garlic cloves, crushed
- 3 tablespoons tomato paste
- 1 tablespoon chopped cilantro
- ¼ teaspoon cayenne pepper
- 1 teaspoon cumin
- 1 teaspoon paprika
- ¼ teaspoon black pepper

Directions
Preheat your oven to 450 degrees and grease a baking dish.

In a saucepan, combine millet and water and bring to a gentle boil; lower heat and simmer for about 15 minutes or until water is absorbed.

In a skillet set over medium heat, heat olive oil and cook on red onion and garlic for about 5 minutes or until tender; stir in ground beef and cook for about 10 minutes or until browned. Stir in cayenne, cumin, tomato paste, paprika and black pepper and cook for 5 minutes.

Stir in the cooked millet and cilantro until well combined; spoon into the bell peppers and arrange them in the greased baking dish; bake in the preheated oven for about 20 minutes or until pepper are tender.

Nutritional Information per Serving:
Calories: 325; Total Fat: 1.4 g; Net Carbs: 28 g; Dietary Fiber: 5.2 g; Sugars: 8.7 g; Protein: 22.3 g; Cholesterol: 51 mg; Sodium: 60 mg

71. Sweet Spiced Mango-Mint Lassi

Yield: 3 Servings
Total Time: 5 Minutes
Prep Time: 5 Minutes
Cook Time: N/A

Ingredients

- 2 cups nonfat Greek yogurt
- 1 large mango, diced
- 1 tablespoon lime juice
- 1 teaspoon ground cardamom
- 1 teaspoon ground star anise
- 2 tablespoons fresh mint
- 2 teaspoons raw honey
- 3 sprigs fresh mint

Directions

Combine all ingredients in a blender and blend until very smooth. Serve garnished with mint.

Nutritional Info per Serving:

Calories: 228; Total Fat: 3 g; Carbs: 43.6 g; Dietary Fiber: 2.1 g; Sugars: 40 g; Protein: 9.4 g; Cholesterol: 10 mg; Sodium: 121 mg

72. Crispy Lemon- Chili Roasted Kale

Yield: 2 Servings
Total Time: 30 Minutes
Prep Time: 10 Minutes
Cook Time: 20 Minutes

Ingredients

- 2 bunches kale, ribs and stems removed, roughly chopped
- 2 tablespoons lemon juice
- 1 teaspoon extra-virgin olive oil
- 1 teaspoon lemon salt
- 2 teaspoons chili powder
- Parmesan wedge

Directions

Preheat oven to 250°F. In a large bowl, massage together kale, lemon juice, extra virgin olive oil, lemon salt and chili powder until kale is tender; spread the kale on a baking sheet and bake for about 20 minutes or until crisp tender. Remove from oven and sprinkle with parmesan cheese. Serve warm.

Nutrition info Per Serving:

Calories: 165; Total Fat: 4.6 g; Carbs: 8.7 g; Dietary Fiber: 2 g; Sugars: 0.5 g; Protein: 2.4 g; Cholesterol: 0 mg; Sodium: 58 mg

73. Low-Carb Cassava Crepes

Yield: 4 Servings
Total Time: 25 Minutes
Prep Time: 10 Minutes
Cook Time: 15 Minutes

Ingredients

- 1 ⅓ cups cassava flour
- 2 egg whites
- 1 cup almond milk
- 2 teaspoons lemon juice
- 2 tablespoons melted coconut oil
- 1 teaspoon stevia
- 1 pinch salt

Directions

In a bowl, whisk together egg whites, almond milk, lemon juice, oil, stevia and sea salt; gradually whisk in cassava flour until well blended and very smooth.

Preheat a nonstick pan and spread in about a quarter cup of batter to cover the bottom. Cook for about 3 minutes per side or until golden brown. Repeat with the remaining batter. Serve with a cup of tea or a glass of juice.

74. Spiced Apple Crisps

Yield: 4 Servings
Total Time: 35 Minutes
Prep Time: 1 Minutes
Cook Time: 25 Minutes

Ingredients

- 4 apples, slices
- 3 tablespoons raw honey
- ½ teaspoon sea salt
- 2 teaspoon cinnamon
- 1 tablespoon virgin olive oil
- 1 teaspoon black pepper

Directions

In a large bowl, stir together cinnamon, raw honey, black pepper and sea salt until well blended; add the apple slices into the mixture and toss to coat well.

Heat olive oil in a skillet over medium heat; add in the apple slices and deep fry until golden browned. Drain the apple crisps onto paper towel lined plates and serve with a cup of tea.

Nutritional Information per Serving:
Calories: 413 Total Fat: 6.3 g; Net Carbs: 26 g; Dietary Fiber: 6.8 g; Sugars: 22.3 g; Protein: 3.9 g; Cholesterol: 0 mg; Sodium: 321 mg

75. Vinegar & Salt Kale Chips

Yield: 2 Servings
Total Time: 22 Minutes
Prep Time: 10 Minutes
Cook Time: 12 Minutes

Ingredients

- 1 head kale, chopped
- 1 teaspoon extra virgin olive oil
- 1 tablespoon apple cider vinegar
- ½ teaspoon sea salt

Directions

Place kale in a bowl and drizzle with vinegar and extra virgin olive oil; sprinkle with salt and massage the ingredients with hands.

Spread the kale out onto two paper-lined baking sheets and bake at 375°F for about 12 minutes or until crispy.
Let cool for about 10 minutes before serving.

Nutritional Information per Serving:
Calories: 152; Total Fat: 8.2 g; Net Carbs: 13.2 g; Dietary Fiber: 2 g; Sugars: trace; Protein: 4 g; Cholesterol: 0 mg; Sodium: 1066 mg

76. Chia Seed Millet Flour Cake

Yield: 16 Servings
Total Time: 50 Minutes
Prep Time: 20 Minutes
Cook Time: 30 Minutes

Ingredients:

- 1 cup vanilla almond milk
- 1 banana, mashed
- 1 tsp. liquid stevia
- ¼ cup fresh lemon juice
- Zest of 1 small lemon
- 1 tbsp. chia seeds
- 1 tsp. vanilla
- ¼ cup millet flour
- ¼ cup coconut flour
- 2 tbsp. corn starch
- ½ tsp. baking soda
- 1 tsp. baking powder
- ½ tsp. cinnamon

Directions

Preheat oven to 350°F.

Coat a 9-inch pie plate with coconut oil.

In a bowl, mix together almond milk, mashed banana, stevia, lemon juice, lemon zest, chia seeds, and vanilla extract.

In another bowl, whisk millet flour, coconut flour, cornstarch, baking soda, baking powder, and cinnamon; stir in the wet ingredients until well blended; transfer to the prepared pie plate and bake for about 30 minutes.

Let cool before serving.

Nutritional Information per Serving:

Calories: 120; Total Fat: 8.3 g; Net Carbs: 9.8 g; Dietary Fiber: 1.8 g; Sugars: 3.2 g; Protein: 1.5 g; Cholesterol: 0 mg; Sodium: 87 mg

DRINKS

77. Spiced Ginger Citrus Juice

Yield: 2 Servings
Total Time: 2 Minutes
Prep Time: 2 Minutes

Ingredients:

- 2 grapefruit
- 2 oranges
- 2 lemons
- 2 tablespoon apple cider vinegar
- 1 cup hot water
- 1-inch fresh ginger
- 1 dash cayenne pepper
- ¼ teaspoon cinnamon

Directions:

Mix together all ingredients and serve warm.

Nutritional Information per Serving:
Calories: 19; Total Fat: 0.3 g; Carbs: 2.2 g; Dietary Fiber: 0.6 g; Sugars: 0.8 g; Protein: 0.4 g; Cholesterol: 0 mg; Sodium: 15 mg

78. Ginger Citrus Asparagus Body Cleanser

Yield: 1 Serving
Prep Time: 10 Minutes

Ingredients

- 1 lime
- 1 lemon
- A bunch of asparagus
- 2 carrots
- 1-piece ginger
- 4 leaves kale
- 2 stalks celery

Directions

Add all ingredients to the juicer and juice. Enjoy!

Nutritional Information per Serving:

Calories: 294; Total Fat: 1.2 g; Carbs: 76.1 g; Dietary Fiber: 14.6 g; Sugars: 48.4 g; Protein: 4.9 g; Cholesterol: 0 mg; Sodium: 85 mg

79. Red Detox Juice

Yields: 1 serving
Prep Time: 10 Minutes

Ingredients

- 1 cup diced watermelon
- 1 beetroot
- 1 lemon peeled
- 1 cup spinach
- 2-inch knob ginger
- 2 kale leaves
- 1 cucumber, chopped
- 2 celery stalks, chopped
- Handful of fresh parsley or cilantro

Directions

Add all ingredients to the juicer and juice. Serve right away.

Nutritional Information per Serving:

Calories: 158; Total Fat: 1 g; Carbs: 39 g; Dietary Fiber: 9 g; Sugars: 20 g; Protein: 5 g; Cholesterol: 0 mg; Sodium: 112 mg

80. Hot Ginger Cucumber & Beet Juice

Yield: 1 Serving
Prep Time: 10 Minutes

Ingredients

- 1 cucumber
- 1 lemon
- 2 carrots
- 1 beet
- 1 clove of garlic
- 1 knob ginger
- 1 raw jalapeño pepper

Directions

Rinse and juice all ingredients. Stir and serve right away.

Nutritional info per Serving:

Calories: 171; Total Fat: 0.9 g; Carbs: 41.4 g; Dietary Fiber: 8.7 g; Sugars: 21.1 g; Protein: 5.8 g; Cholesterol: 0 mg; Sodium: 169 mg

81. Apple & Citrus Beet Juice

Yield: 2 Servings
Prep Time: 5 Minutes

Ingredients

- 3 beetroots
- 2 medium apples
- 2 carrots
- 2 oranges, peeled
- 2 lemons, peeled

Directions

Wash and juice everything. Enjoy!

Nutritional info per Serving:

Calories: 310; Total Fat: 1.1 g; Carbs: 78.8 g; Dietary Fiber: 15.9 g; Sugars: 56.8 g; Protein: 6 g; Cholesterol: 0 mg; Sodium: 161 mg

82. Celery Pineapple Juice

Yield: 1 Serving
Prep Time: 10 Minutes

Ingredients

- 2 slices of pineapple
- 3 large organic celery stalks
- 1 piece of fresh gingerroot
- 1 piece of fresh turmeric root
- 3 sprigs of parsley

Directions

Wash and juice everything. Enjoy!

Nutritional info per Serving:

Calories: 41; Total Fat: 0.3 g; Carbs: 9.2g; Dietary Fiber: 2.6 g; Sugars: 5.7 g; Protein: 1.1 g; Cholesterol: 0 mg; Sodium: 98 mg

83. Kale & Apple Juice

Yield: 2 Servings
Prep Time: 10 Minutes

Ingredients:

- 2 leaves kale
- 2-inch piece of fresh ginger
- 1 apple
- 2 medium carrots
- 1 lemon
- 2 celery stalks
- 1 large beet

Directions

Rinse and peel your ingredients and then slice into pieces; run through the juicer. Serve chilled. Enjoy!

Nutritional info per Serving:
Calories: 131; Total Fat: 0.5 g; Carbs: 32.6 g; Dietary Fiber: 6.7 g; Sugars: 19.7 g; Protein: 2.7 g; Cholesterol: 0 mg; Sodium: 103 mg

84. Refreshing Cucumber Citrus Juice

Yield: 2 Servings
Prep Time: 10 Minutes

Ingredients

- ½ cucumber, peeled
- 1 orange, halved and peeled
- ½ lemon, peeled
- 1 apple
- 2-inch piece of ginger
- 4 carrots
- 1 tablespoon raw honey

Directions

Rinse the ingredients and juice them all! Stir in a tablespoon of raw honey to sweeten the juice. Serve chilled.

Nutritional info per Serving:
Calories: 205; Total Fat: 0.5 g; Carbs: 52.2 g; Dietary Fiber: 8.9 g; Sugars: 36.6 g; Protein: 3 g; Cholesterol: 0 mg; Sodium: 88 mg

85. Cucumber Aloe Vera Drink

Yield: 2 Servings
Prep Time: 10 Minutes

Ingredients

- 1/2 Aloe Vera leaf
- 1/2 pineapple, cored
- 1/2 lemon
- 1 small cucumber
- 1 cup coconut water

Directions

Wash veggies and fruits.

Slit the edges of aloe vera with a knife to open the outer layer; scoop out the gel and set aside.
Run all ingredients through a juicer and stir in aloe vera gel and coconut water. Serve right away.

Nutritional info per Serving:
Calories: 140; Total Fat: 1 g; Carbs: 33.4 g; Dietary Fiber: 6.1 g; Sugars: 20.1 g; Protein: 4.5 g; Cholesterol: 0 mg; Sodium: 260 mg

86. Berry Freshness

Yield: 4 Servings
Prep Time: 10 Minutes

Ingredients

- 4 lemons
- 2-inch piece of fresh ginger root
- 1 cup strawberries
- 1 cup raspberries
- 1 cup blueberries
- 1 cup blackberries

Directions

Rinse the ingredients and juice them all! Stir in a tablespoon of raw honey to sweeten the juice. Serve chilled.

Nutritional info per Serving:

Calories: 84; Total Fat: 0.9 g; Carbs: 21.2 g; Dietary Fiber: 7.2 g; Sugars: 10 g; Protein: 2.1 g; Cholesterol: 0 mg; Sodium: 3 mg

87. Carrot & Celery Juice

Yield: 2 Servings
Prep Time: 10 Minutes

Ingredients

- 1 grapefruit
- 2 oranges
- 2 tomatoes
- 6 medium carrots
- 2 stalks celery
- A pinch of cayenne pepper

Directions

Wash fruits and veggies. Peel and section grapefruit and oranges. Run everything through a juicer. Stir in cayenne and serve chilled.

Nutritional info per Serving:
Calories: 207; Total Fat: 0.6 g; Carbs: 50.1 g; Dietary Fiber: 11.4 g; Sugars: 34.1 g; Protein: 4.8 g; Cholesterol: 0 mg; Sodium: 146 mg

88. Ginger Berry Pineapple Drink

Yield: 2 Servings
Prep Time: 10 Minutes

Ingredients

- 1-inch slice of fresh turmeric or ginger
- 1 cup blueberries
- 1 cup diced pineapple
- 4 celery ribs
- 1 cup fresh parsley
- 1 cup mint leaves

Directions

Wash and juice everything. Enjoy!

Nutritional Information per Serving:

Calories: 136; Total Fat: 1.2 g; Carbs: 31.3 g; Dietary Fiber: 8.6 g; Sugars: 16.7 g; Protein: 4.2 g; Cholesterol: 0 mg; Sodium: 97 mg

89. Gingery Apple & Spinach Juice

Yield: 1 Serving

Prep Time: 10 Minutes

Ingredients

- 1-inch slice of ginger
- 1 apple
- 3 carrots
- 1 cup mint leaves
- 1 cup cilantro

Directions

Rinse all the ingredients and run them through a juicer. Serve right away.

Nutritional Information per Serving:

Calories: 121; Total Fat: 0.3 g; Carbs: 29.2 g; Dietary Fiber: 8.3 g; Sugars: 16.3 g; Protein: 2.8 g; Cholesterol: 0 mg; Sodium: 82 mg

90. Chilled Pineapple-Ginger Ale

Yield: 2 Servings
Prep Time: 10 Minutes

Ingredients

- 1-inch slice of ginger
- 1 cup diced fresh pineapple
- 1 cup spinach
- 1 cup purple cabbage

Directions

Wash and juice everything. Serve chilled.

Nutritional Information per Serving:
Calories: 57; Total Fat: 0.3 g; Carbs: 14 g; Dietary Fiber: 2.4 g; Sugars: 9.4 g; Protein: 1.4 g; Cholesterol: 0 mg; Sodium: 19 mg

91. Citrus Ginger Beet Juice

Yields: 2 servings
Prep Time: 10 Minutes

Ingredients

- 2 beets
- 1 tangerine
- 1 orange
- 1 lime
- 2 carrots
- 2 cups dandelion greens
- 2-inch knob ginger

Directions

Add all ingredients to the juicer and juice. Enjoy!

Nutritional info per Serving:

Calories: 173; Total Fat: 0.9 g; Carbs: 41.6 g; Dietary Fiber: 9.4 g; Sugars: 25.1 g; Protein: 5.2 g; Cholesterol: 0 mg; Sodium: 163 mg

92. Super Green Detox Juice

Yield: 2 Servings
Prep Time: 10 Minutes

Ingredients

- 1 apple
- 1 cup seedless grapes
- 1 lemon
- 2-inch ginger root
- 1 cup pineapple
- 1 cucumber
- 1/2 cup parsley
- 2 mint sprigs

Directions

Add all ingredients to the juicer and juice. Enjoy!

Nutritional Information per Serving:
Calories: 158; Total Fat: 0.8 g; Carbs: 35.6 g; Dietary Fiber: 5.5 g; Sugars: 30 g; Protein: 2.4 g; Cholesterol: 0 mg; Sodium: 15 mg

93. Refreshing Kiwi Cucumber Drink

Yields: 2 servings
Prep Time: 10 Minutes

Ingredients

- 4 carrots
- 1 cup sprouts
- 1-cm fresh ginger
- 1 kiwi fruit
- 1 lemon
- 1 green apple
- 1 cucumber
- 2 stalks celery
- 1 cup parsley

Directions

Add all ingredients to the juicer and juice. Enjoy!

Nutritional Information per Serving:
Calories: 173; Total Fat: 0.8 g; Carbs: 42.3 g; Dietary Fiber: 9.5 g; Sugars: 23.8 g; Protein: 1.4 g; Cholesterol: 0 mg; Sodium: 126 mg

94. Ginger Cabbage Drink

Yield: 1 Serving
Prep Time: 10 Minutes

Ingredients

- 1/4 medium pineapple
- 1 lemon, peeled
- 1-inch fresh ginger
- 2 large cucumbers
- 1 cup chopped cabbage
- ½ cup fresh mint

Directions

Juice all the ingredients, one at a time, in a juicer and serve.

Nutritional Information per Serving:
Calories: 125; Total Fat: 0.8 g; Carbs: 30.2 g; Dietary Fiber: 7.4 g; Sugars: 10.5 g; Protein: 5.1 g; Cholesterol: 0 mg; Sodium: 46 mg

95. Cleansing Kale Juice

Yield: 1 Serving
Prep Time: 10 Minutes

Ingredients

- 1/2 cup chopped kale
- 1/2 cup baby spinach
- 1 cucumber
- 1-inch ginger
- 2 carrots
- 1 pear
- 1/2 apple
- 2 celery stalks

Directions

Add all ingredients to the juicer and juice. Enjoy!

Nutritional Information per Serving:
Calories: 259; Total Fat: 0.8 g; Carbs: 64.6 g; Dietary Fiber: 12.9 g; Sugars: 36.7 g; Protein: 5.4 g; Cholesterol: 0 mg; Sodium: 160 mg

96. Ultimate Ginger Apple Cleanser

Yields: 1 Serving
Prep Time: 15 Minutes

Ingredients:

- 1 organic beet, peeled
- ½ organic lemon, peeled
- ½ inch ginger root
- 2 organic red apples, chopped
- 3 organic carrots, peeled
- 6 organic kale leaves
- 1 cup chopped cabbage

Directions:

Place all the ingredients in a juicer and juice. Stir to mix well and serve with ice cubes.

Nutritional info per Serving:
Calories: 232; Total Fat: 0.6 g; Carbs: 57.4 g; Dietary Fiber:11.2 g; Sugars: 33.2 g; Protein: 5.4 g; Cholesterol: 0 mg; Sodium: 147 mg

97. Ginger Celery & Apple Drink

Yield: 1 Serving
Prep Time: 10 Minutes

Ingredients

- 1 lemon
- 1/2 green apple
- 1 cups spinach
- 1 radish
- 2 stalks celery
- 1.5-cm ginger
- ½ cup parsley

Directions

Add all ingredients to the juicer and juice. Enjoy!

Nutritional Information per Serving:
Calories: 150; Total Fat: 0.2 g; Carbs: 36.7 g; Dietary Fiber: 8.7 g; Sugars: 9.1 g; Protein: 5.7 g; Cholesterol: 0 mg; Sodium: 100 mg

98. Ginger Citrus Detox Juice

Yield: 1 Serving
Prep Time: 10 Minutes

Ingredients

- 1 lemon, peeled
- 1-inch knob fresh ginger root, finely grated
- 1 orange, peeled
- 1 grapefruit, peeled
- 1 garlic clove
- A pinch of cayenne pepper

Directions

Juice all the ingredients in a juicer, except cayenne pepper; stir in cayenne pepper and serve.

Nutritional Information per Serving:

Calories: 11; Total Fat: 0 g; Carbs: 0 g; Dietary Fiber: 0 g; Sugars: 1 g; Protein: 5 g; Cholesterol: 0 mg; Sodium: 2 mg

99. Ginger Pineapple Reboot Juice

Yield: 1 Serving
Prep Time: 10 Minutes

Ingredients

- 1 pineapple center
- 1-inch ginger root
- 2 carrots
- 3 celery stalks
- Handful mint leaves
- Small handful of cilantro

Directions

Juice all the ingredients in a juicer and serve.

Nutritional info per Serving:

Calories: 152; Total Fat: 0.5 g; Carbs: 37.2 g; Dietary Fiber: 6.8 g; Sugars: 23.3 g; Protein: 2.8 g; Cholesterol: 0 mg; Sodium: 137 mg

100. Super System Cleanser Drink

Yield: 1 Serving
Prep Time: 10 Minutes

Ingredients

- ¼ cup fresh aloe vera juice
- 1 lemon, peeled
- 5 asparagus spears
- 1 cucumber
- 1 carrot
- 10 stalks celery
- Handful of cilantro
- Handful of parsley

Directions

Add all ingredients to the juicer and juice. Enjoy!

Nutritional Information per Serving:

Calories: 113; Total Fat: 0.9 g; Carbs: 26.1 g; Dietary Fiber: 8.4 g; Sugars: 11 g; Protein: 6.4 g; Cholesterol: 0 mg; Sodium: 160 mg

101. Healthy Beet Juice

Yield: 1 Serving
Prep Time: 10 Minutes

Ingredients

- 1 medium carrot
- 1 cucumber
- 1 orange, peeled
- 1/2 cup cranberries
- 1 large beet
- Ice cubes

Directions

Juice everything in a juicer except ice cubes; stir in ice cubes and enjoy!

Nutritional Information per Serving:

Calories: 412; Total Fat: 1.6 g; Carbs: 91.4 g; Dietary Fiber: 18.5 g; Sugars: 64.8 g; Protein: 8 g; Cholesterol: 0 mg; Sodium: 167 mg

101. Ginger Celery and Cucumber Detoxifier

Yield: 1 Serving
Prep Time: 10 Minutes

Ingredients

- 1 (1-inch) pieces ginger root
- 1 lime, peeled
- 1 orange
- 1 cucumber
- 1 beet
- 2 stalks celery
- 1/2 medium apple

Directions

Add all ingredients to the juicer and juice. Enjoy!

Nutritional Information per Serving:
Calories: 136; Total Fat: 0.8 g; Carbs: 35.5 g; Dietary Fiber: 7.3 g; Sugars: 18.4 g; Protein: 3.8 g; Cholesterol: 0 mg; Sodium: 59 mg

Conclusion

The human body as made in such a way that it could take of all its vital processes such as digestion on its own without outside help. It was so efficiently designed that it could fix any problem with any of its organs without outside intervention.

Unfortunately, with the evolution of what we eat from what our ancestors ate has rendered the body incapable of keeping up with all its processes without breaking down.

This book explores one vital organ and what it is responsible for, what affects it and ways in which we can be able to keep it healthy. The first step is going back to the diet that was followed by our ancestors. As simple as eating healthy and natural foods. Feed your body with food that will nourish it and not make it seek.

Am confident that you have been able to get important information on how to keep your pancreas healthy and how to manage any symptom of pancreatitis. Enjoy the recipes on our food section that have been specifically designed to help you manage and prevent symptoms of pancreatitis.

Remember to share with friends and family so we are able to help so many people who are living in the anguish of pancreatitis pain.

All the best as you embrace a healthier life that is now more informed!

Made in United States
North Haven, CT
08 December 2023

45367499R00072